THE BABY
CHECKUP BOOK

Other books by these authors:

Sheilah Hillman
    Public Relations for Private Schools
    Traveling Healthy:
        A Complete Guide to Medical Services in 23 Countries

Robert S. Hillman, M.D., F.A.C.P.
    The Red Cell Manual
    Traveling Healthy:
        A Complete Guide to Medical Services in 23 Countries
    Clinical Skills:
        Interviewing, History Taking and Physical Diagnosis

James H. Moller, M.D., F.A.A.P.
    Congenital Heart Disease
    Essentials of Pediatric Cardiology
    Heart Disease in Infants
    Clinical Skills:
        Interviewing, History Taking and Physical Diagnosis

THE BABY CHECKUP BOOK
A Parents' Guide to Well Baby Care

SHEILAH HILLMAN

James H. Moller, M.D., F.A.A.P. and Robert S. Hillman, M.D., F.A.C.P., consultants, with a foreword by R. Don Blim, M.D., F.A.A.P. past president of the American Academy of Pediatrics

Bantam Books
Toronto • New York • London • Sydney

THE BABY CHECKUP BOOK: A Parent's Guide to Well Baby Care
A Bantam Book / June 1982

ACKNOWLEDGMENTS
*Photographs and drawings pages 25, 27, 28, 33, 37, 39, 46, 82, 84, 90, 96 from
Clinical Skills by Robert S. Hillman et al. Copyright © 1981 by McGraw-Hill
Inc. Used with the permission of McGraw-Hill Book Company.
NCHS Growth Charts reprinted by permission of the National Center of
Health Statistics. Courtesy of Ross Laboratories, Columbus, Ohio.*

Library of Congress Cataloging in Publication Data

Hillman, Sheilah.
The baby checkup book.

Bibliography
1. Infants—Care and hygiene.   I. Title.
RJ61.H56   649'.122   81-70919
ISBN 0-553-01398-X   AACR2

Published simultaneously in the United States and Canada

PRINTED IN THE UNITED STATES OF AMERICA

0 9 8 7 6 5 4 3 2 1

To Adam, Gregory,
Anna, Eric, Justin,
Wayne, Derek, Jennifer, Elizabeth,
Laura, David, and Clara

CONTENTS

FOREWORD

Children are our greatest natural resource, and caring for these children—parenting—bestows the greatest challenge, responsibility, and opportunity that one ever assumes. The importance of a child's first years cannot be emphasized enough.

After more than twenty-five years in pediatric practice, I believe I have developed a perspective on parenting that comes neither naturally nor easily to most parents. Parents should have some understanding and appreciation of this unique individual called a newborn. The prospective mother needs to learn about those factors that have a major impact on the newborn, factors such as maternal health, nutrition, and medication. The decisions a mother makes about herself—whether to smoke, to consume alcohol, to provide herself with proper nutrition—bear a tremendous relevance for her child. The exact nature of the exciting birth process, the vital first examination, the importance of the first feeding, the infant's first few days, and the developmental milestones must all demand the attention of the new parents. Parents should realize some basic facts, principles, guidelines, and recommendations about children while simultaneously recognizing that there is a great deal of variation from the norm and a great deal of flexibility in dealing with the newborn.

In addition to the awareness of the parents concerning their child is their awareness of the triangular relationship formed between themselves, their child, and the pediatrician. To provide the best health care for the infant, it is essential that the parents and the pediatrician develop a working partnership; each is able to provide different elements of care that must combine to form an effective effort dedicated to the welfare of the newborn. The pediatrician must be well trained, knowledgeable, and compassionate. The parents, for their part, need to be as well informed as possible.

The Baby Checkup Book addresses my concerns and offers parents an excellent foundation upon which to build. Presenting information in an organized sequential fashion that is consistent with the practice patterns of most pediatricians, it describes the normal newborn and its development. And in emphasizing issues such as immunization, accident prevention, preventive health care, and anticipatory guidance, it performs a much needed service to any parents who give it their attention. Indeed, everyone—children and physicians as well as parents—will benefit from this thoughtful book.

R. Don Blim, M.D., F.A.A.P.
President, American Academy of Pediatrics, 1980-81

ACKNOWLEDGMENT

I would like to thank the health professionals listed below for their help in the preparation of this book. What is even more remarkable than their expertise is their willingness to share it with others.

Mary Andrews, R.P.T., University of Washington Child Development and Mental Retardation Center, Seattle

Robin Beck, M.D., University of Washington Family Medicine Clinic, Seattle

Fay Benjamin, Washington State Parents Anonymous

Cynthia Branson, S.T., M.A., University of Washington Child Development and Mental Retardation Center, Seattle

Diana Breithaupt, P.N.P., University of Washington Pediatric Clinic, Seattle

Kenneth Feldman, M.D., Odessa Brown Children's Clinic, Seattle

Kristin Hardwick, B.S., R.D.H., University of Washington Child Development and Mental Retardation Center, Seattle

Sandra Griffiths, M.D., University of Washington Pediatric Clinic

Katie Hicks, R.N., Washington State Traffic Safety Commission

Ruth Little, Sc.D., director, University of Washington Alcohol and Drug Abuse Institute, Seattle

Richard W. Moriarity, M.D., director, National Poison Center Network, Pittsburgh

Connie Nakao, R.N., M.N., University of Washington Child Development and Mental Retardation Center, Seattle

Lois Neu, P.N.P., M.S.N., University of Washington Child Development and Mental Retardation Center, Seattle

Peggy Pipes, R.D., M.P.H., University of Washington Child Development and Mental Retardation Center, Seattle

Debbie Richards, Washington state chairperson, Action for Child Transportation Safety

Robert Scherz, M.D., Mary Bridge Child Health Care Center, Tacoma

David Shinn, director, Office of Public Education, American Academy of Pediatrics

Robert Telzrow, M.D., formerly University of Washington Pediatric Clinic, Seattle

Special thanks to Dr. Gordon E. Pyne, Sandpoint Way Medical Center, Seattle, my children's pediatrician for sixteen years, and to Sharon Swanson, the special pediatric nurse who makes his office run like a fine Swiss watch.

INTRODUCTION

The well baby care program you choose for your newborn is one of the most important decisions you'll ever make. In partnership with the pediatrician, clinic, or family medicine practitioner of your choice, you'll be giving your baby the best possible start in life and guaranteeing the healthiest of possible futures.

The ideal time to choose your baby's doctor is before the baby is born. For recommendations, ask your friends who have children or call your local county medical society for the names of pediatricians in your area. Then visit some doctors. Some parents interview three to five doctors before making their choice. Some doctors charge for these pre-care interviews and some do not.

Remember that you may be seeing your baby's doctor regularly for as long as eighteen years, the age at which many pediatricians turn their patients over to "adult" physicians. That means you not only need to respect the doctor for his or her skill and reputation, but that you ought to like him or her as a person as well. Your personalities should be, if not a match, at least not a complete mismatch. If you're a relaxed, communicative kind of person, you will not be happy with a rigid, authoritarian physician. The reverse is also true. So tell the doctor what kind of person you are and what kind of relationship you hope to have.

As important as the doctor you choose is the location of the office and the way it is run. Is it located conveniently near you? Is there plenty of parking, and is the parking free? Most important, how efficiently is the office run? Do patients consistently wait for a long time to see the doctor? (For the answer to that one, ask the people in the waiting room.) In well-run offices, patients are rarely kept waiting for more than a few minutes, and this kind of efficiency is not that difficult to achieve. Very simply, doctors who are committed to well-run offices have them.

If cost is a consideration, be sure to talk to the doctors about it. Ask what their fees are. No child in the United States need be denied a regular health-care program on the basis of lack of funds. In every community there are well baby clinics that charge only what parents are able to pay. These clinics are usually associated with teaching hospitals, children's hospitals, and community service programs.

No matter what health-care program you choose for your child, it is almost certain to be greatly influenced by the American Academy of Pediatrics. An organization of board-certified pediatricians, the AAP figures prominently in this book, just as it ultimately will in the health of your child. This is because much of the child care practiced in the United States today is based on AAP recommendations. The academy appoints standing committees to research thoroughly and make recommendations about a number of health topics critical to good patient care—nutrition, breast-feeding, and immunizations, to name a few. Committee findings are constantly reviewed, updated, and made available to pediatricians and well baby clinics across the country.

In the first two years of life, your baby will have several scheduled visits to the doctor. The number varies from doctor to doctor. The AAP recommends that babies be seen at least five times during the first year of life and at least three times during the second.

The Baby Checkup Book is organized just like your baby's visits to the doctor or clinic. Every well baby checkup has four components—a physical examination, special procedures (shots, tests), discussion of parent concerns, and anticipatory guidance (things the parents should be alert for in the weeks to come). Every well baby checkup chapter in this book is organized the same way—a description of the physical examination, an explanation of the special procedures, discussion of parent concerns, and anticipatory guidance (called "Reminders" throughout the book).

In a clinical setting, babies are not always seen by a physician but by medical students, pediatric nurse practitioners (PNPs), and other physician's assistants who are responsible for key parts of the checkup. For the sake of convenience, however, this book refers to the person conducting the examination as *doctor, pediatrician,* or *examiner.*

1
THE NEWBORN
THE FIRST
FEW MINUTES

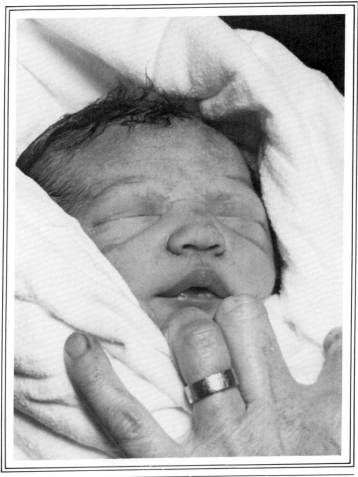

✓ CHECKLIST

DELIVERY-ROOM PROCEDURES

_____ Apgar evaluation at age one minute: _____

_____ Apgar evaluation at age five minutes: _____

_____ Brief physical examination

_____ Weigh and measure

    Weight _____

    Height _____

    Head circumference (OFC) _____

    Chest circumference _____

_____ Attach identification tags to wrist and ankle

_____ Instill silver nitrate in eyes

_____ Clamp cord

_____ Take sample of cord blood (optional)

_____ Estimate gestational age

_____ Give injection of vitamin K (optional)

The first few minutes of life are critical for your baby. He arrives wet, cooling off fast, his nose, mouth, and throat clogged with fluid and debris from the womb. He also arrives to face a challenging environment. This has nothing to do with the fact that the lights in the delivery room are bright, the temperature is somewhat cool, and the first hands to touch him are more efficient than loving. It is because he has lived for forty weeks in an airless, temperature-controlled environment where everything he needed for his existence was provided. Now he must adapt to quite a different environment. Suddenly he must be able to do for himself things he's never had to do before— breathe air, adjust and control his own body temperature, take nourishment, and eliminate waste.

The team of doctors and nurses in the delivery room is specially trained to help the baby over the first hurdles and monitor his progress through the first few minutes of life. They begin to help him breathe before he is even born, suctioning his nose and mouth as his head appears and continuing until he is breathing well on his own.

At the very moment of birth, your baby gets his first physical "checkup." At age one minute, he is observed closely by delivery-room personnel and then rated for his performance on five items—heart rate, breathing, general appearance, muscle tone, and the response to a gentle stimulus such as a flick on the sole of his foot or a tickle in one nostril. He gets two points for each perfect item.

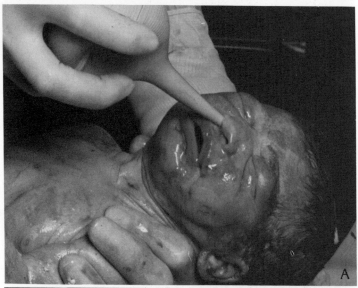

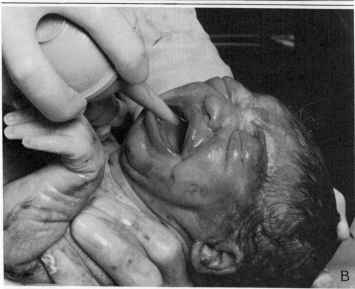

*During birth and immediately after,
the newborn's nose (A) and mouth (B) are
suctioned to help him breathe on his own.*

Called the Apgar score, this evaluation of his condition at birth is repeated again when he is five minutes old. It was developed by and named for the late Dr. Virginia Apgar of New York's Columbia Presbyterian Medical Center and is performed by most hospitals in the United States and some hospitals abroad as well. Doctor Apgar, an anesthesiologist who assisted at hundreds of births, noticed striking differences in the conditions of newborns and developed her evaluation as a way of describing them and relating them to the effects of maternal anesthesia. Today the score is used as a guideline to a baby's immediate needs in the delivery room and as a way of following his progress through the first few minutes of life. The Apgar score is also used as a measure of recovery from the birth process.

APGAR SCORE*

Signs	0	1	2
Heart rate/ pulse	none	below 100 beats per minute	above 100 beats per minute
Breathing	none	slow, irregular	cry
Muscle tone	limp	some movement of extremities	physically active
Response to stimulus	none	grimace	cry
Appearance/ color	blue or pale	extremities blue, body pale	pink

*Adapted from Apgar, V.: *Current Researches in Anesthesia and Analgesia,* 32–260, 1953.

Heart Rate/Pulse The baby's heart rate—the number of times his heart beats per minute—is determined by listening to his heart with a stethoscope. The heart of a healthy newborn beats more than 100 times a minute.

Below 100 beats a minute indicates the infant is in some distress and requires further observation.

Breathing   Clearing the baby's airway—his nose and breathing passages—is the doctor's first concern. Mucus and debris from the womb are gently sucked from his nose with a rubber-bulb syringe. Often this is done while the baby is still in the process of being born, when only his head has appeared. If a baby doesn't breathe on his own soon after his nose has been suctioned, he receives a zero on the Apgar scale. If his breathing is slow and irregular, he is given a score of 1. If he is breathing well and crying lustily, he gets a 2 for breathing.

Muscle Tone   In scoring a newborn, attention is paid to the baby's muscle tone. A limp, floppy baby gets no points, scoring zero. A baby who keeps his arms and legs tucked in (flexed) close to his body and who is also able to move them vigorously gets a high score of 2.

Response to Stimulus   Once the baby is breathing and his heart is beating, he is checked to see how he responds to stimulation from the environment. Sometimes a soft rubber tube is placed in one of his nostrils, or the doctor or nurse flicks the sole of his foot with a finger. Irritated, the baby should either make a face (grimace) or cry because of the disturbance. He gets 1 point for grimacing, 2 points for crying, no points for no response.

Appearance/Color   Pink all over is the healthiest color for a newborn to be because it indicates plenty of oxygen is circulating throughout his body. In black babies, the inside of the mouth, palms of the hands, and soles of the feet are checked for pinkness. If a baby is pale or blue, it means that he is oxygen-starved and that his lungs aren't getting enough oxygen to his extremities. Most babies arrive looking a bit blue (cyanotic) but gradually turn to a healthy pink color within the first five to ten minutes.

Although the Apgar score does *not* predict the future, the five-minute score does reflect the newborn's general condition and provides guidelines for further delivery-room care and observation. A score of 9 or 10 is excellent, and 7 or better is considered normal. A lower score means that

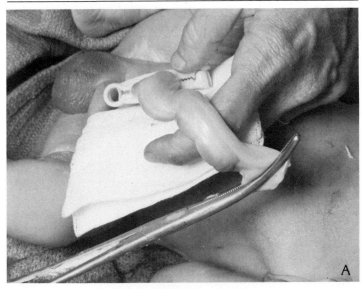

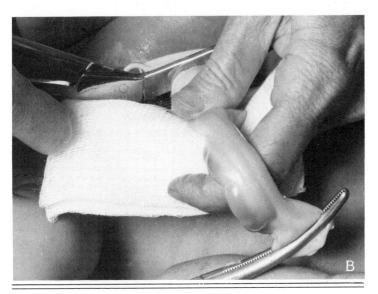

*The doctor first clamps (A) and then
cuts (B) the umbilical cord. Note the coating
of vernix caseosa on the baby's leg (C), (next page).*

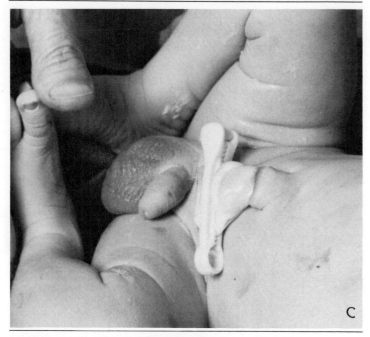

C

the baby was in some distress at the time of birth, but it doesn't necessarily mean that he is seriously impaired. A *very* low score, however, particularly at five minutes, may indicate a birth defect or other serious problem.

There was a time when Apgar scores were not routinely shared with parents. It was perhaps too scary to tell them that their newborn was having some difficulty and too easy for parents to predict a glum future for their child based on the Apgar score. Now, however, many parents want to know everything there is to know about their babies, and a number of obstetricians consider it their obligation to share the information with parents who request it.

Once the umbilical cord is clamped, the baby is dried off, wrapped in a blanket, and placed either under a radiant heat source or on top of a heated pad. In some hospitals the newborn heat source is known affectionately as the "bun warmer." It is important to a newborn's good health that his body temperature be maintained at a normal level. For their size and weight, newborns have three times as much skin surface as an adult and far less protective fat. Because of their large surface area compared to weight, babies are like little radiators. They lose body heat fast—four times faster than a grownup, and that's why it's so important to keep them warm.

After the baby is dry, warm, breathing on his own, and the Apgar score has been determined, he's given a quick physical examination to rule out any obvious defects. The doctor begins by looking at the skin. Newborn skin is covered with vernix caseosa, a cheesy, white, somewhat sticky substance. Some babies are born with more of it than others, and it is believed that this substance may provide some kind of necessary protection to the skin in the first few days of life. Because of this belief, there is a growing trend of patting the baby dry in the delivery room rather than giving him a bath. The skin is often covered, too, with

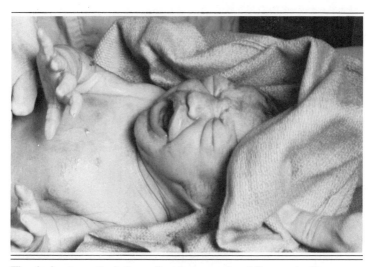

The baby is patted dry, allowing much of the protective coating of vernix caseosa to remain on the skin.

lanugo, a fine, downy hair that usually disappears within a week or two.

The brief physical examination performed in the delivery room is done to determine that the baby is normal, that the size of his head is about right—not too large (an indication of hydrocephalus, or water on the brain) and not too small (an indication of microcephaly, or an undeveloped brain)—that eyes, ears, nose and mouth are present; that there are two arms and two legs that seem to match up to their mates in size and shape; that there are five fingers and five toes on each hand and foot with no webbing in between; that there are no obvious sinuses (holes) along the body surface where there are supposed to be none; and that by contrast there *are* holes where they are expected—that the anus is patent (open), for example.

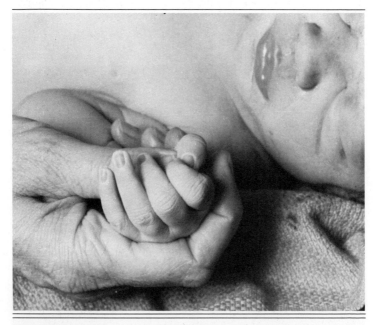

The doctor performs a brief physical examination to check that the most obvious things are normal—that the baby has the right number of fingers and toes, for example.

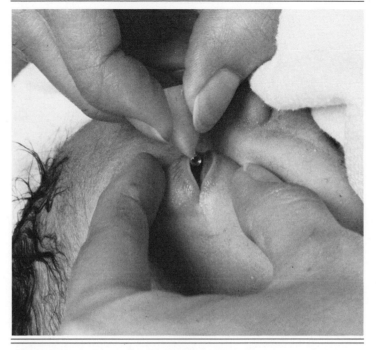

*A drop of weak silver nitrate solution is placed in
each of the baby's eyes to prevent infection.*

A drop of weak silver nitrate solution is placed in each
eye to prevent infection. Sometimes drops or ointment
containing either Tetracycline or Erythromycin are used
instead of the silver nitrate. They are less irritating to the
baby's eyes. In most cases it isn't possible for parents to
make the choice concerning which agent is used in the
baby's eyes. Although silver nitrate has proved useful in
controlling eye infections, some parents fear that the resulting irritation—temporary swelling of the eyelids and conjunctivitis (reddening and irritation of the eye)—interferes
with bonding. Bonding is the familiarization process that
begins to take place between parent and child, beginning in
the first few minutes of life, and much of it depends on the
baby's being able to see the parent, something he can't do

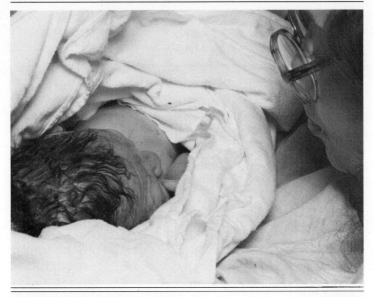

*Eye contact between mother and
baby begins just minutes after birth and is
important to the bonding process.*

very well if his eyes are swollen shut by the silver nitrate. On the other hand, the silver nitrate is important because it counteracts any eye infection the baby may have contracted while passing through the birth canal. Such infections are serious and can cause blindness.

An injection of vitamin K to prevent common bleeding complications has been considered good delivery-room procedure, although its effectiveness is being challenged and may result in a change of policy in some hospitals. A sample of blood may be taken from the umbilical cord, then refrigerated and stored in case any blood tests need to be done. This procedure is optional and is performed at the discretion of individual hospitals.

Next the baby is weighed and measured. The baby is usually placed on the scales wrapped in a blanket to keep him warm. The weight of the blanket is, of course, deducted to determine his true birth weight. The average baby weighs 7½ pounds, and boys are slightly heavier than girls. Ninety-five percent of all babies weigh between 5½ and 10 pounds, with premature babies usually, but not always, weighing less than full-term ones.

In some hospitals, measurements are taken in the delivery room, although they may also be taken later in the nursery. The length of the average newborn is 20 inches, with the range of normal between 18 and 22 inches . . . and growing! Each new generation steadily exceeds the previous one by one inch. The average head circumference of a newborn is 14 inches, or 34–35 cm. Birth length is not an indication of future adult height.

Before your baby leaves the delivery room, identification bands are placed on his wrist and ankle. In some hospitals, foot-, palm-, and fingerprints are taken as well, for the hospital is as eager as you are that you take the right baby home with you.

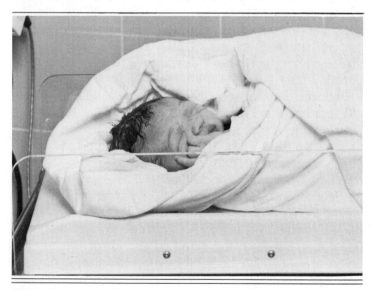

The baby is weighed wrapped in blankets to keep him warm. Heat loss is dangerous for a newborn.

Another delivery-room procedure is to determine your baby's gestational age, that is, how old he was when he was born. Was he a full-term baby, was he a little bit premature, or was he perhaps post-term, or late by a few days? Full-term babies are born 280 days (40 weeks) from the first day of their mother's last normal menstrual period. Babies born before 37 weeks are considered premature, or preterm, and have to be watched carefully for signs of the complications associated with premature birth—breathing troubles, increased susceptibility to infection, jaundice, and anemia; and instability of body temperature, among others.

Babies born prematurely are often called preemies by the public, but *preterm* is the term more often used now by health professionals. When a baby is born prematurely, his early arrival has to be taken into consideration for some time to come. He is literally a baby longer because things happen to him later. It is important to continually adjust and correct for the amount of his prematurity, especially in the first year and a half of life. The average baby walks at age one year, for example, but the baby who was born four weeks prematurely is more likely to walk at age 13 months—one year plus a four-week allowance for his premature birth. Corrections for the premature baby are particularly important where developmental milestones are concerned.

Some of the observations necessary to determine how old your baby really is can be done as soon as he is born. Others concern the nervous system and must be delayed until he is at least 48 hours old so there will be no lingering effects from any anesthesia used in the delivery. There are a number of indications of gestational age—everything from the presence of breast tissue and the firmness of ear cartilage to the number of creases in the soles of the feet. There are standard forms that doctors can use to estimate gestational age. Some of the items on the forms are complicated. They measure fairly esoteric neurological signs such as the precise angle at which the infant holds his wrist with manipulation. Others, though, are easy enough for parents to observe for themselves.

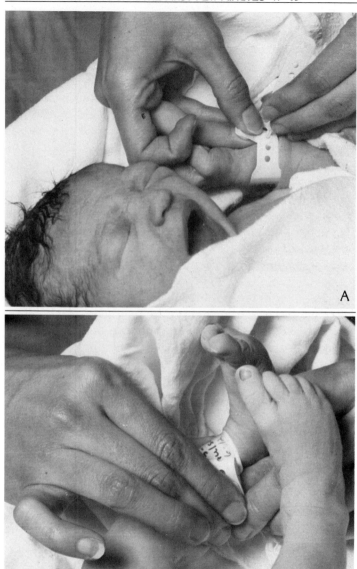

Before the baby leaves the delivery room, identification bands are placed on his wrist (A) and ankle (B).

Hair A baby's hair at term grows in silky strands, which it began to do at 38 weeks. Before that, it is downy, like the lanugo that covers a newborn's skin. The post-term baby has little or no lanugo on his skin.

Breast The presence of breast tissue indicates that a baby is full-term. The doctor feels the breasts to make this determination. If there is fat tissue under and around the nipple, the baby is full-term. The breasts of full-term babies are slightly raised; those of premature babies are flat. The areola, the pigmented area around the nipples, is enlarged in post-term babies.

Skin The skin of a healthy full-term baby is pink and opaque, and the blood vessels beneath the surface of the skin cannot be seen. The skin of a premature baby, on the other hand, is thinner and more transparent. The large vessels beneath can be seen through the skin. The skin of post-term babies is leathery, cracked, and wrinkled.

Feet Full-term babies have creases on the soles of their feet that extend downward to their heels. Babies born earlier have creases that cover about two-thirds of the foot but don't reach the heel. Still earlier, there are only one or two creases on the sole of the foot.

Ears The ears of a full-term baby are firm to the touch. When folded, they spring quickly back into place. The more premature a baby is, the softer is the ear and the less rapidly it springs back into position.

Genitals/Male A sign of a full 40-week gestation in male babies is that the testicles are large and descended and the scrotum deeply creased. The creases are called rugae. When boys are premature, their testicles may be undescended or descended with only a few rugae, depending on the degree of prematurity.

Genitals/Female Female genitals at term are completely covered by the labia majora, the outer skin folds. In premature girls, the labia minora (inner folds) and clitoris show to varying degrees, depending on the amount of time the baby is premature.

It is very important to know a baby's gestational age. Sometimes babies are born who appear to have a normal birthweight but who are actually premature by one or more weeks when their gestational age is calculated. Such a baby would show signs that are normal for premature babies—descreased response to the environment, difficulty feeding, irregular sleep patterns, and unusual body postures and changes in the color of the skin. If the baby had been mistaken for a full-term newborn on the basis of his relatively heavy birthweight, all of those symptoms might easily be wrongly diagnosed as evidence of defect or disease. By correctly establishing gestational age, errors like this, resulting in needless worry to both doctors and parents, can be avoided.

In forty weeks your baby has grown and developed from a single fertilized cell too small to be seen with the naked eye to a fully formed person with functioning organ systems. This growth and development, astonishing by any standards, continues at breakneck pace after birth as well. From the standpoint of development, birth is really just a minor event in the continuing process of building a human being. Before he was born, you were able to influence profoundly your baby's growth and development by the care you took of yourself during pregnancy. Now that he is born, you can continue to give him the best possible start in life. How your baby grows and flourishes after birth will depend not only on his genetic endowment—the actual physical and mental traits he inherited from you—but upon the loving, caring environment you provide for him as well.

PARENT CONCERNS

Every parent in the world shares the same concern seconds after the birth of a child: Is my baby okay: Is he healthy and perfectly formed? Miraculously the answer is usually yes. About 90 percent of newborns are indeed perfect. The percentage goes even higher if you include as normal and healthy (and almost perfect) those babies born with insignificant and common defects such as an extra tag of skin near the earlobe.

2
THE NEWBORN
THE FIRST
FEW HOURS

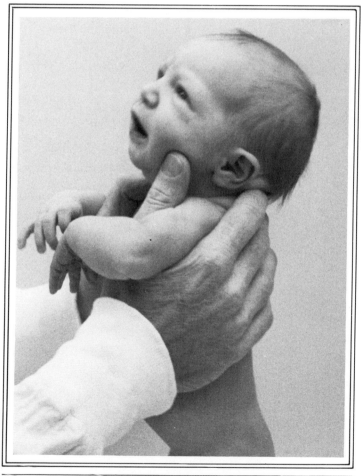

✓ CHECKLIST

NURSERY PROCEDURES

Complete physical examination
(within 24 hours of birth)

_____ Head	_____ Feet
_____ Neck	_____ Hips
_____ Arms and underarms	_____ Femoral pulses in the groin
_____ Hands	_____ Genitals
_____ Abdomen	_____ Back and spine
_____ Legs	_____ Anus

WITH INSTRUMENTS

_____ Heart	_____ Nose
_____ Lungs	_____ Mouth and throat
_____ Eyes	_____ Ears

Complete Neurological examination
(24 hours before discharge from hospital)

_____ Test reflexes (blinking, hearing, patellar/knee jerk, palmar grasp, plantar grasp, rooting, sucking, prone, placing, stepping and Moro/startle)

_____ Examine eyes

_____ Perform transillumination of the skull

So here she is, Ms. America. Only a few hours old, she already knows how to move her head to avoid smothering, how to search for and suck vigorously on a nipple, how to "walk," step up over an obstacle, and grab your finger and hold on tightly. She also knows how to protect her eyes from bright lights and to protest strenuously against things that startle her. Not bad for a beginner.

Unless she is rooming in with you, your baby will spend the first hours of her life in the hospital nursery. Because the first six hours continue to be critical, the staff in the nursery takes their job seriously, which explains why the nurses sometimes seem to act as if the baby is theirs as much as yours. The staff does not usually welcome intrusions into their domain from anybody—not Mom, not Dad, not the grandparents, and not even a staff physician who doesn't have permission to be there. For those six hours, the nurses monitor your baby closely, watching her breathing and color, taking her vital signs such as temperature and heart rate, and being sure she remains stable and in no distress.

After about four hours, if the rectal temperature remains stable and everything continues to look good, a nurse gives the baby her first bath and shampoo. The bath will probably be a dry one that includes only a swabbing off with sterile water and patting dry. This is to preserve the baby's protective coating (vernix caseosa). The dry method also avoids the problem of cooling the body off too much, a continuing concern with newborns. Then the baby is dressed and fed three to four teaspoons of water, after which she is swaddled and placed in her bassinet. There her temperature, heart rate, breathing, and general level of activity continue to be monitored.

Within 24 hours of birth, your baby will be given an extensive physical examination that will set the standard for all future checkups she will have in the first two years of life. Sometimes parents are permitted to see this examination, so be sure to let your doctor know if you're interested.

The following examination description tells only part of the story. Chapter 4 has further details and photographs of the physical examination.

THE NEWBORN PHYSICAL EXAMINATION

First the doctor washes his hands and forearms thoroughly to protect the baby from infection, the most feared enemy of a hospital nursery. Babies are an easy target for infection. Not only do they have an open wound (the umbilical stump), but they also have had little experience coping with the bacteria we all carry on our skin and in our mouths. So, depending on nursery procedure, the doctor may also be required to wear a sterile gown, gloves, and mask for the examination. He tries to choose a time between feedings when your baby is not hungry enough to be fussy, but not so well fed that she is very sleepy and lethargic. If she becomes cranky during the exam, he will quiet her with a pacifier or with the tip of a well-scrubbed finger.

General Appearance   It's tough getting born sometimes. Babies can bruise their heads and break their collarbones in the process. Their tender skin may be injured by instruments used to aid in the delivery. Babies born by Caesarean section have their share of woes, too. They escape the bruising journey down the birth canal, but they are snatched unceremoniously from their waiting place, usually at least a few days prematurely. Fortunately, birth injuries are not very high, only about 2 to 7 in every 1,000 births.

Before doing anything, the doctor simply looks at and

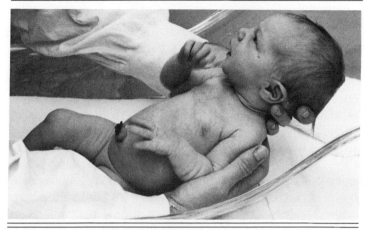

The doctor begins the examination simply by observing the baby.

listens to the baby for a bit. A baby signals that she is healthy and normal in many ways, and the doctor can read these signs just by looking at her. So that is the way the examination begins. One sign of a normal, healthy baby is the way she holds her body when she's lying on her back. She keeps her arms and legs flexed (folded) in toward her body when she's at rest. When she moves her extremities, she does so vigorously and symmetrically, so that there is equal range of movement on both sides of her body. She lies on her stomach with her head turned to one side, her pelvis high, and her knees drawn up under her tummy. She keeps her fists closed, with the thumbs visible and not tucked into the palms of her hand.

As the newborn breathes, her belly moves in and out with each breath, and she breathes easily without making wheezing or grunting sounds. And when she cries, it is a healthy, lusty cry. Crying that is hoarse or too low or too high in pitch signals an abnormality, as does no crying at all.

Undressing the baby, the doctor notes her body proportions, the condition of her skin, and whether there are any birth injuries or defects. He is also looking for rashes and birthmarks. It is normal for the skin of some newborns to be scaly and peeling at first. It becomes smooth by itself in a week or two. Normal skin may also be wrinkled and loose. This is because only 28 percent of a baby's weight at birth is fat. In the first few months of life, babies lay down more fat, which takes up any slack in the skin that existed at birth.

It is also normal for the hands and feet to be somewhat purplish in color because of sluggish circulation, which will self-correct with time. Until the baby is better able to adjust her own body temperature, it isn't unusual, either, for her skin to appear mottled at times in response to temperature changes in the environment. Sometimes a baby even shows a harlequin phenomenon, in which half her body becomes blue while the other half remains a normal color. Alarming to parents, it's not dangerous for the baby.

As for rashes and birthmarks, two of the most common rashes have uncommon names. One is milia. Almost half of all newborns have milia over their noses. Pimply in appearance, this is just a slight swelling of the child's normal oil glands. It goes away without treatment. Similarly, half of all full-term newborns have a blotchy red rash with yellowish blisters called erythema toxicum. This rash, which can appear almost anywhere on the body and cover an extensive area, appears in the first two days of life and disappears without treatment in another two days.

Among the most common birthmarks are cafe au lait spots, hemangiomas, and Mongolian spots. Cafe au lait spots are light, coffee-colored, and permanent. They occur most frequently on the trunk and extremities. There are several kinds of hemangiomas, the most common being flat ones—small, pale pink patches that commonly appear on the upper eyelids, between the eyes, and on the upper lip and the nape of the neck. They usually fade completely in one or two years. Mongolian spots are grayish-blue spots found mostly in black and Oriental babies, less commonly in whites. They are usually seen on the trunk, buttocks, and lower extremities, rarely on the face. They usually disappear on their own in the first few years of life.

Included in this assessment of your baby's general appearance may be some of the most minute details imaginable, such as the pattern of hair on her head, its distribution and length, the pattern of creases on the palms of her hands and the tips of her fingers, the symmetry of her facial features, and the position of her ears. There are normal and abnormal characteristics for each of these items and many more.

Chest (Thorax) When the doctor examines a newborn's chest with the stethoscope, he is checking both the

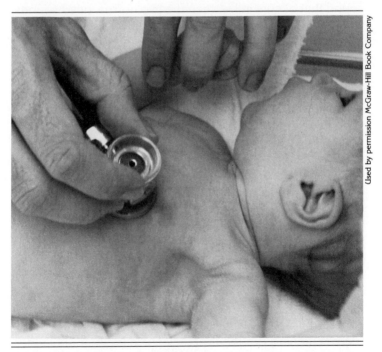

The doctor listens to the newborn's chest with a stethoscope, both for heartbeat and for sounds of breathing.

heart and lungs. It may take some time to perform this part of the examination.

The chest wall is round—later it becomes more cylindrical in shape—and breathing is mostly abdominal. Even so, the doctor can check the chest to be sure it expands evenly on both sides, an indication that both lungs are filling to the same capacity.

The breathing rate should be about 30 or 40 breaths a minute, slower than the rate at birth, which was 60. Irregular breathing is normal in the first few days of life, especially in premature babies.

With his stethoscope, the doctor listens to the baby's heart. The pulse rate in normal newborns is between 120 and 160 beats per minute, faster than the adult rate of 60 to 90. Sometimes the doctor hears a murmur, a swishing sound that occurs in between the two normal heart sounds, *lub* and *dup*. Such temporary murmurs, also called transient or innocent, are found in as many as half of all newborns but usually disappear in the first 24 to 48 hours of life. Nevertheless, babies with murmurs are observed carefully in the next few hours so that a specialist can be called in for a consult, should the murmur not disappear on schedule. Murmurs associated with more serious, congenital heart disease don't usually appear until later, when the baby is a few weeks old.

The breasts of both boys and girls may be temporarily enlarged at birth and may also leak a fluid called witch's milk. Caused by estrogen levels received from the mother, the condition is temporary and harmless. It usually disappears by the time the baby is 2 or 3 months old.

Stomach (Abdomen) The doctor inspects the umbilical cord stump for irritation, bleeding, or discharge. Yellow (meconium) staining of the cord is an indication of fetal distress at the time of birth. With the pads of his fingers, the doctor gently probes (palpates) the lower abdomen, searching out the liver, spleen, kidneys, and bladder. He checks to be sure they are the proper size and not swollen by disease. He is also making certain there are no foreign masses or tumors in the belly area.

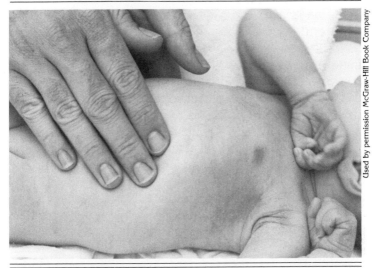

With the pads of his fingers, the doctor gently probes (palpates) the lower abdomen, searching out the liver, spleen, kidneys, and bladder.

Genitals (External Genitalia)   The genitals of baby girls are usually enlarged at birth, caused by loss of estrogen hormone from the mother. There may also be a slightly bloody discharge from the vagina for the same reason. This is normal and will disappear.

The genitals of baby boys who have had a breach birth (bottom first) may be swollen but will reduce to normal size in a few days. The doctor feels the scrotum for testes, which may be present either there or further up in the inguinal canal. The foreskin is not retractable at birth, a condition that can persist to age one year and beyond in uncircumcised males.

In both sexes, the doctor identifies the urethral opening, through which the baby urinates. If the baby urinates during the exam—and little boys frequently do—the doctor will observe the stream. A healthy boy can shoot up to 18 inches into the air. Less spectacular, but just as healthy, is the 2-to-3-inch arc of a baby girl.

Hands and Arms Normally, new babies keep their arms and legs folded in toward their bodies, with their hands closed into fists. In the beginning, they like to stay curled up as if they were in the womb. If you gently straighten out an arm or leg, it acts like a little rubber band and quickly springs back to its original position. This is called the recoil reflex and is normal.

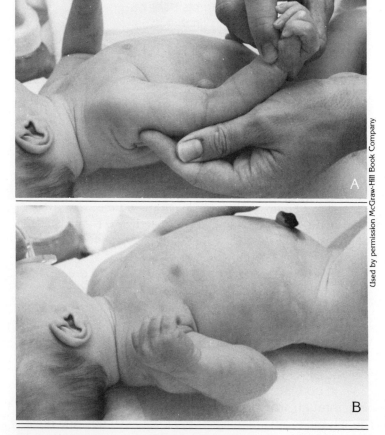

Used by permission McGraw-Hill Book Company

The doctor gently stretches out the baby's arm (A), which springs back to its original position (B) upon release. This is called the recoil reflex.

The doctor checks the hands for normal crease patterns in the palms and for color. Pale fingers can signal a circulatory problem or anemia. He also feels under the baby's arms, checking for enlarged lymph nodes, a sign of infection or tumor.

Feet, Legs and Hips The newborn examination is the same as described in Chapter 4.

Spine and Back When the doctor turns the baby over to inspect her back and spine with his fingers, she will automatically turn her head to one side to avoid smothering. It is reassuring for parents to know that normal babies can't suffocate when lying on their stomachs. It is one of the many reflexes all newborns have for self-preservation. Others are described later in this chapter, in the newborn neurological examination.

The doctor listens to the baby's lungs again with the stethoscope. He can hear the air going through the passages and can tell if there is fluid in the lungs. There should not be. He listens to her breathing and can tell if any sounds are abnormal. He also examines her spine and tailbone

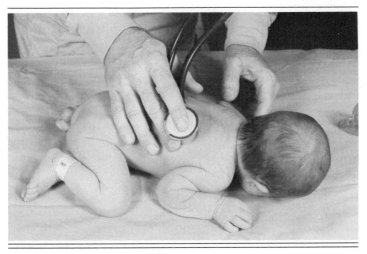

With the baby on her tummy, the doctor listens to the lungs.

(coccyx) for tufts of hair, dimples, growths, or openings that would indicate a spinal malformation.

Head Turning the baby onto her back again, the doctor checks her head and face carefully. He is looking to see if everything is reasonably symmetrical or whether her features are abnormally lopsided. Nobody's perfect, of course, but there are some features—eyes set too far apart, ears set too low—that signal recognized abnormalities.

The head is also examined for molding, caput, and cephalhematoma. Molding is a temporary reshaping of the head as it passes through the birth canal. Caput is a swelling and bruising of the soft tissue. Cephalhematoma is a soft bump caused by bleeding under the scalp. All of these conditions go away by themselves without treatment.

The skull of a newborn is made of partially calcified bony plates that fit together loosely like a jigsaw puzzle with missing pieces. The missing pieces are the fontanels, little skin-covered spaces that give the bony plates room to expand and allow the brain to grow, something it will do a considerable amount of in the first year of life.

The anterior fontanel, the one at the top front of the baby's skull, is normally soft and flat when the baby is held upright. It shouldn't bulge outward or be depressed inward. In some babies, the soft spot pulsates slightly. This is normal. Reasonable care must be taken of the soft spots, although it is hard to injure them, short of dropping the baby on her head. The routine head examination is described further and the fontanels are illustrated in Chapter 4.

Neck Newborns have short necks, which grow longer as the child gets older and the spine grows. Sometimes a newborn's head tilts to one side because of injury at birth to muscles in the neck. Called torticollis, this condition is usually temporary and self-correcting.

The doctor feels both sides of the neck, checking for enlarged lymph nodes and an enlarged thyroid, also for size, suppleness, and freedom of movement. He also checks the collarbone, or clavicle, to be sure it wasn't fractured during birth.

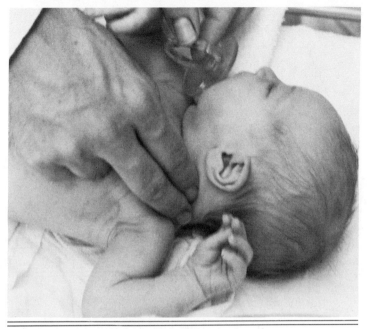

*The doctor feels the neck carefully
for thyroid and lymph-node enlargement.*

Mouth With a penlight, the doctor examines the mouth and tongue, ruling out cleft palate or other abnormalities in the structure of the mouth. He also inspects the gums and any teeth present at birth. Such teeth, called milk teeth, are rare and usually fall out before the first teeth come in.

Sometimes there are little white cysts, called Epstein's pearls, on the gums. They disappear by themselves in a few months. The frenulum is the connective tissue under the tongue. Sometimes it extends almost to the tip of the tongue, a condition called tongue tie. There is no treatment required, for it does no harm and does not result in a speech impediment. Newborns don't have much saliva. The amount increases later, at about the time teething begins.

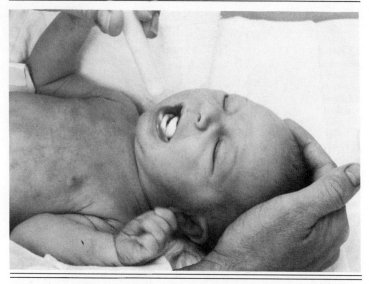

*With a penlight, the doctor
examines the mouth and tongue.*

Throat   The throats of newborns are hard to examine, but it is usually possible to see the uvula, the tag at
the back center of the throat. A uvula split into two pieces
(bivalve) is abnormal. Tonsils are not visible in a newborn.

By moving the tongue blade back further into the
baby's mouth, the doctor makes her gag for just a split
second. This is the way he tests to be sure cranial nerves IX
and X are working properly. If the baby gags, it means she is
capable of swallowing.

Nose   A baby's nose humidifies the air she breathes
and also traps bacteria and harmful materials in a continually moving blanket of mucus. Babies can only breathe
through their noses and not through their mouths, so it's
essential that the nasal passages be clear. The doctor
closes first one nostril and then the other, observing
breathing. If a newborn has trouble breathing through one
nostril or another, it might mean there is still birth debris in
the nasal passages or that the baby has narrow passages.

Ears The doctor notes the position, shape, and firmness of the outer ears (pinnas). Using the otoscope, he can confirm that the ear canal is open (patent) but can't usually see the eardrum because the passage is frequently filled with vernix caseosa, the same substance that covers the baby's skin at birth.

There is evidence that babies can hear from about the twenty-sixth week of pregnancy. In trying to determine whether or not a newborn can hear, the doctor takes into consideration the family history and whether or not the mother had during pregnancy a disease such as German measles that affects an unborn baby's hearing. Newborns normally demonstrate their ability to hear by startling when they hear a noise. If there is a suspected hearing loss, a newborn can be referred to an audiologist, a hearing specialist, for evaluation. Although there are tests that can be administered to small babies, the true extent of hearing loss can't accurately be established until a child is older.

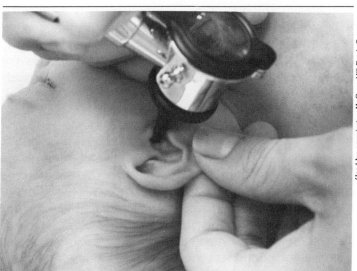

Used by permission McGraw-Hill Book Company

The doctor uses an otoscope to confirm that the newborn's ear canal is well formed and open.

Eyes   Unlike other organs, the eyes are almost fully grown at birth, already three-quarters of their adult size. The iris, or colored part, has less color at birth than it will later. Final eye color develops in the first year of life. Often babies have no tears until they are about four months old.

Newborns are able to focus and see best at a distance of about 8 inches (20 cm), just about the distance to their mother's faces at feeding time. They pay attention to (attend to) faces and objects for only brief periods at first, but their attention span increases as they get older.

In trying to determine how well your baby sees, the doctor will consider the family history—how well the parents see and whether or not the mother had German measles during pregnancy, which could have adversely affected the baby's eyesight.

A newborn's eyes are difficult to examine. Often they are irritated and bloodshot, the lids puffy from the silver nitrate drops instilled at birth. The newborn understandably keeps them tightly shut, but the doctor is usually able to perform the examination described in the next chapter.

Measurements   Finally, the doctor measures the baby's head at the level of the eyebrows with either a paper or cloth tape and records it on a growth chart like the one provided at the back of this book. He also measures the chest circumference at the level of the nipples and records it as well.

THE NEWBORN
NEUROLOGICAL EXAMINATION

Just before you bring your baby home—some time between 48 and 72 hours after birth—she will have a complete neurological examination to be sure that her nervous system is working properly and that she seems to see and hear. By testing her responses to external stimuli, one by one, the doctor checks out the delicate circuitry of her brain and spinal cord, much as a television repairman tests the circuitry of a TV set. Think of it as a quick check of the wiring.

Most of the examination is designed to test reflexes, involuntary actions all humans have when stimulated in different ways. A normal reflex shows a normal "circuit." If, for example, you shine a light into the baby's eyes and she blinks, it means she can see. It also means she was trying to protect herself from the light. That's what reflexes are all about—they're an emergency device that shortens the body's time response to dangerous, threatening, or annoying situations.

There are plenty of things to check out in a baby, even though the brain is still undeveloped and has limited function. In a single year it will grow to 82 percent of its adult size.

Some reflexes, such as the knee jerk, persist throughout life, but many—the palmar, plantar, and sucking reflexes—disappear until old age, and others disappear forever. An example of one of the vanishing ones is the little-known Badkins reflex. If you press firmly into the palms of a newborn, her mouth opens. Following are

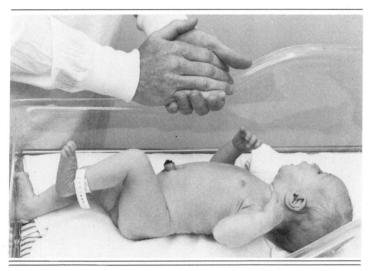

When a newborn hears a loud noise, such as clapping, she startles. This indicates that she can hear.

some, not all, of the reflexes seen in normal newborns. During the actual examination, all of these, and more, are tested.

Blinking Reflex   Your baby blinks both eyes when a light is shined on one eye, even if the lids are closed. This means that she can see, that the impulse to the brain was received and an attempt was made to shut it out.

Hearing Reflex   When your baby hears a loud noise, such as a clapping sound, near her ear, she startles. This means she can hear.

Palmar Grasp Reflex   If you place your finger into the palm of your baby's hand, she will grasp your finger. If you then pull your finger up and away from the baby, she will hold on tightly. Sometimes you can even lift her a bit off the examining table. She is clinging to protect herself from falling.

Plantar Grasp Reflex   If you put your thumb in the sole of your baby's foot and press just under the toes, they

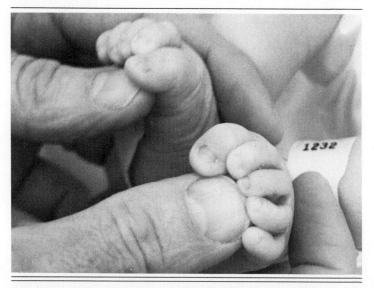

*When the doctor presses his thumbs into the
soles of the newborn's feet, the toes curl downward in
a grasping motion called the plantar grasp reflex.*

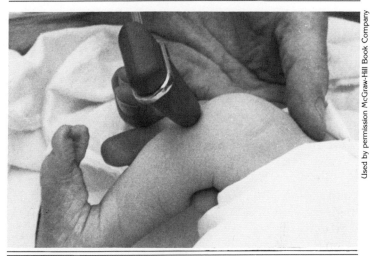

Tapped lightly with a rubber hammer,
the baby's knee jerks. This is called the patellar reflex.

will normally curl downward around your thumb. It is a gripping, clinging reflex much like the palmar grasp.

Patellar Reflex   Tapped lightly with a small rubber hammer, the baby's knee jerks in a reflex action. The motion should be brisk and symmetrical, proof of normal nerve pathways.

Rooting Reflex   If you brush your baby's cheek at the corner of the mouth with your finger, she will turn toward it, looking for a nipple.

Sucking Reflex   If you place your finger or a pacifier in the baby's mouth, she will suck on it. Strong sucking is necessary for survival, so the doctor must evalute it during this examination.

Prone Reflex   Placed face-down on her stomach, your baby should move her head to one side or the other to avoid smothering.

Stepping Reflex   When your baby is held upright, leaning slightly forward with her feet touching a surface, she makes walking movements.

Placing Reflex When your baby is picked up under the arms and the instep of one foot is placed under the edge of a table so that it touches, she lifts her foot and puts it on top of the table.

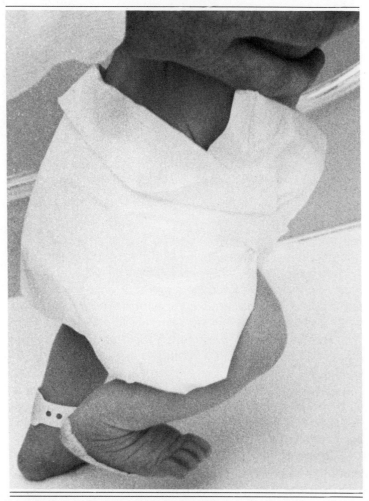

When a newborn is held upright, leaning slightly forward with her feet touching a surface, she makes walking movements. This is called the stepping reflex.

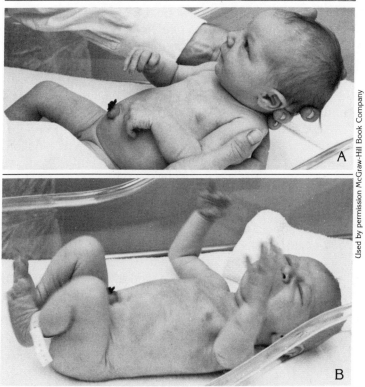

Used by permission McGraw-Hill Book Company

*To test the Moro (startle) reflex, the doctor first
lifts the baby's head and upper torso a bit (A) and
then allows it to fall back (B). Startled, the
baby throws out her arms as if to hug something.*

Moro (Startle) Reflex   Testing this reflex, and some
of the others as well, is best left to the doctor. Your baby is
placed on her back. Her head and upper back are lifted up a
bit, then allowed to fall back. She isn't hurt, but she *is*
startled. Her arms fly out as if to hug something, and her
hands open from their usual closed-fist position. Then she
kicks her legs and (usually) has a good cry. Sometimes
babies startle spontaneously while both awake and asleep.
Some also startle regularly when they are moved or burped.
They don't always cry at the end of every startle.

Extremities   Newborns hold themselves naturally in a position with their arms and legs coiled toward their bodies, as described earlier in this chapter. The examiner straightens out an arm and then lets go, watching to see that it recoils to its original position. He does the same with the other arm and with the legs. Then he flexes the baby's hands and feet to check their mobility and range of motion.

Eyes and Head   The eyes and head are thoroughly examined as part of the newborn neurological examination. As the baby's head is moved up and down and left to right, the position of her eyes should stay straight ahead like a doll's eyes. In fact, it's called the doll's-eyes reflex. Also, the pupils of her eyes should narrow when stimulated by light, and she should turn her head toward a soft light. The doctor also checks for the red reflex described in Chapter 4, in the section entitled "The Eyes."

Your baby is taken into a darkened room where a special shielded flashlight is held against her head for a

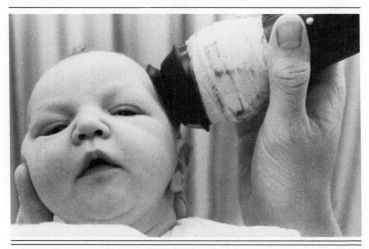

The doctor uses a special shielded flashlight to see inside the baby's head and determine whether there is abnormal blood or fluid over the brain. This is called transillumination of the skull.

procedure called transillumination of the skull. It allows the doctor to see whether there is blood or fluid over the brain.

THE PKU TEST

Toward the end of your hospital stay, when the baby has been fed milk for at least 24 hours, a few drops of blood will be taken from her heel with a sterile needle and sent to the hospital laboratory to be tested for phenylketonuria (PKU). This is the rare inability of some babies to metabolize a common substance called phenylalanine, found in milk and meat products. The condition, which occurs in only one of about every 14,000 births, can be corrected by means of a special formula and diet if it is discovered early. Otherwise, affected babies suffer brain damage and mental retardation from the buildup of abnormal amounts of phenylalanine in their blood.

A PKU test performed before the baby is 72 hours old is not completely accurate, but some hospitals are forced to do them because babies frequently go home before the third day. If your baby's PKU screening test was done before the third day, or if it wasn't done at all, it should be done in the doctor's office or clinic when you bring the baby in for her first checkup at age 2 to 4 weeks. You can also make arrangements for the test to be done after discharge at the hospital where the baby was born.

NUTRITION

In an ideal world every baby would be breast-fed. All a baby needs for the first few months of life is milk, and not surprisingly, the most perfect milk for a human infant is mother's milk. Breast-feeding was strongly recommended by the nutrition committees of the American Academy of Pediatrics and the Canadian Paediatric Society in *Breast-Feeding, A Commentary in Celebration of the International Year of the Child, 1979.** Not only is breast milk quality controlled—bacteria-free and at perfect serving

Pediatrics, Vol. 62, No. 4, October 1978.

temperature—but it also appears to provide the newborn infant with immunological advantages.

There is evidence that fewer illnesses are reported in breast-fed babies in the first year of life and that they also have a lower incidence of allergy-related illnesses, such as asthma and eczema, later in life. Breast milk contains antibodies that appear to help protect the newborn against severe intestinal infections as well. And there is increasing evidence that mother's milk helps provide resistance to other diseases while the baby's own immune system is developing. Respiratory infections, meningitis, and infections of the bloodstream have been reported to be less frequent in breast-fed babies.

Another advantage to breast-feeding is that it helps promote bonding between mother and child. There is a natural closeness at feeding time with no impersonal propping of a bottle. The possibility of overfeeding the baby is also greatly reduced when the baby is breast-fed. The breast-fed baby nurses until she is satisfied, and the parents don't have to deal with how many ounces are left in the bottle. There is a tendency for parents to relate empty bottles, and later, clean plates, with good health, when obesity may actually be the result.

But this is the real world, a world where some mothers work and some babies are adopted and where breast-feeding isn't always possible. If you cannot or choose not to breast-feed your baby, there is a variety of commercial formulas available. Most of these are made from modified cow's milk, the exception being those made from soybeans for babies who are allergic to cow's milk.

Just as breast milk is perfect for human babies, cow's milk is perfect for calves, which grow much bigger and faster than babies. Cow's milk has to be altered considerably to make it fit for human infant consumption. The curd (coagulated part) of cow's milk is too tough and has to be softened by heat treatment and homogenization. The indigestible butterfat content has to be replaced with vegetable oils, and in the process most of the cholesterol is removed (but human milk contains cholesterol, which may be important in early feeding). The protein and mineral content has to be reduced, a process that also reduces the number of calories. Cow's milk has to be fortified with vitamins and minerals (different from the ones previously removed). And finally, sugar has to be added to bring the calorie count to 20 per ounce, the same as breast milk.

Infant formulas are available in three forms: ready-to-feed (just open the can and feed the baby the contents), concentrated liquid, and powder (add water before feeding). When water is to be added, the supply has to be potable, or pure enough for drinking, and the amount added must be *exactly* as directed on the label. If too little water is added, the baby gets too rich a mixture, is force-fed, and becomes grossly overweight. If too much water is added to the formula, the baby literally starves from lack of nutrition. Too often parents alter the recommended amount of water, thinking it will somehow benefit the baby, when in fact it is an extremely dangerous practice.

Once you've decided what to feed the baby, let the baby decide how much and how often she wants to eat. Feeding is a baby's very first social experience, in addition to being the most important for survival. It is also the only experience over which babies have any kind of control, and it is healthy for them to be in control of their own feeding situation, within reason, from the very beginning.

Most babies know when they are hungry and how much they want to eat. Creating a schedule around those needs makes the most sense. In the first few weeks some babies are hungry every two or three hours, so you can see how futile it would be to try to feed such infants every four hours. Most parents are quickly able to strike a balance between scheduled feedings and demand feeding, neither of which usually proves exactly right for either baby or parent.

As for how much a baby eats, the baby knows best in most cases. Babies shouldn't need to be coaxed through a certain number of minutes at the breast or a required number of ounces in the bottle. Very simply, they stop eating when they are satisfied, so if they fall asleep or turn their heads away, it means they don't want any more. And, very likely, they don't need any more.

If your baby is bottle-fed, ask the doctor about sterilization. He may not think it is necessary, and a number of well-known institutions in the United States no longer recommend it when the local water supply is known to be pure and dependable. A baby's stomach and intestines, after all, are not germ-free except for the first few hours of life. In some cases, thorough cleaning of bottles and careful preparation of formula can be as effective as sterilization.

Position is an important consideration when feeding a baby. The infant should be held in a semireclining position, never flat on her back. When a baby is fed lying down, milk may be regurgitated through the Eustachian tubes into the middle ear. This leakage is a major cause of ear infections in the first year of life.

PARENT CONCERNS

Before you take your baby home from the hospital, you'll no doubt have many questions. Don't be bashful about asking them of either the nurses or the doctor. Following are just a few of the concerns new parents commonly have.

Bathing and Handling Babies don't need to be bathed daily. Sufficient is a routine of every other day, or even less frequently, with sponges in between and careful attention to the diaper (perianal) area. A girl's genitals require careful cleaning, spreading apart the labia (outer folds) and washing the area within carefully with a soft cloth. A cheesy substance collects there that needs to be cleaned daily. Clean from front to back to avoid contaminating the vaginal area with material from the anal area. *Never leave your baby unattended in the bath, not even for a few seconds.* Don't leave newborns unattended on tabletops, either. Always keep a firm hand on the baby's stomach. Shampoos are necessary no more than twice a week.

Your baby's head is quite big compared to the rest of her, and her neck muscles aren't strong enough yet for her to support her own head. This is called head lag, and it means that whenever she's handled for the first three months or so, her head must be carefully supported until she's strong enough to do it for herself.

Diapering is a common-sense operation. Remove the soiled diaper, clean the genital/anal area thoroughly with plain water and a soft cloth, and put on a fresh diaper so that it is tight enough to stay put, but not so tight to cause discomfort. Powders and lotions are not recommended. Not only are they not necessary, but powders are a health hazard. Used carelessly, they may be inhaled by the baby, causing respiratory illness and even death. Because some baby powder containers resemble nursing bottles, they are also a danger to older children, who try to "drink" them.

Bowel Movements   A newborn's first bowel movement is greenish brown and should occur in the first twelve hours or at birth. The color and slightly sticky consistency are the result of her having drunk amniotic fluid during the last three months of pregnancy. In the next few days, movements are first dark green, then yellow and seedy. By the second or third day, they become soft and yellow. Generally, bowel movements of breast-fed babies are softer than those of babies fed formula.

What kind of diapers you use is up to you. Cloth diapers require laundering but are much less expensive to use than disposable ones. Also, some babies develop rashes because of the plastic portion of disposable diapers. Plastic traps warmth and moisture in the diaper, making it a perfect place for bacteria to grow. Plastic pants may cause the same problem, so whenever possible the baby ought to wear just diapers and no plastic pants. Diapers should be changed as soon as possible after they have been soiled or wet.

Bowlegs   Rare is the newborn who doesn't seem to be bowlegged. Rarer still is the newborn who actually *is* bowlegged. When the baby is on her back, straighten out one of her legs as the doctor does in his first hospital examination. If you can draw an imaginary straight line from the baby's hipbone through the bump on the bone

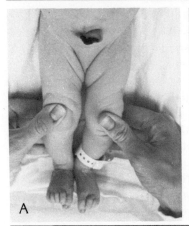
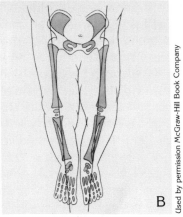

A

B

Although many newborns appear to be bowlegged, few really are. The doctor straightens the legs (A) to check that there is a straight line from the crest of the hipbone through the bump on the bone under the kneecap and down to the bones in the second toe (B).

under the kneecap to her second toe, then her legs are straight. The bowed appearance will correct itself by the time she is 2 to 3 years old.

Circumcision Care In 1971 a committee of the American Academy of Pediatrics reported that there was no longer any medical reason to recommend routine circumcision of baby boys. It remains a matter of individual choice or religious custom, however, and if your baby has been circumcised, you will need to keep his genital area scrupulously clean and dry during the healing process, which will last about eight or ten days. If the doctor recommends keeping a sterile gauze pad over the area, be sure there is plenty of vaseline on the pad to prevent sticking. If there is no pad, a thin coat of vaseline should be applied. Circumcision should not be done before a baby is at least 24 hours old. Low birthweight is a contraindication to circumcision. So are rash, fever, and illness.

Cord (Umbilicus) Care The cord stump should be kept clean and dry. Until it falls off—anywhere from ten days to two or three weeks—babies should have only sponge baths. An alcohol-soaked cotton swab is a good cleaning agent. Any foul smell, discharge, or reddening of the surrounding skin should be reported to the doctor. Sometimes a hernia makes the cord, and later the belly button, stick out. This is common and usually corrects itself by the time the baby is 18 months old. No treatment is required.

Crossed Eyes Newborns are not as efficient at tracking and focusing with their eyes as they will be in the weeks to come. Many seem to have crossed or wandering eyes occasionally. True strabismus, the medical term for crossed eyes, does not become a cause for concern until the baby is 6 months old and continues to have crossed eyes at times. Babies of any age whose eyes appear to be crossed *all* the time should be evaluated by an eye specialist (ophthalmologist).

Jaundice Jaundice is fairly common in newborns. It usually appears in the first two or three days after birth and is recognizable by the yellowish tint it gives to the baby's skin and to the whites of her eyes. When a baby is born, she has lots of extra red blood cells left over from the low-oxygen atmosphere of her mother's womb. These cells need to be broken down by the body into iron, protein, and a yellowish pigment called bilirubin. The pigment needs to be gotten rid of, and this job falls to the liver, which pumps it first into the bile and then into the intestine. Since the baby's liver isn't mature enough yet to handle the load, the excessive amount of yellow pigment in the baby's system shows up in the skin and eyes.

This kind of jaundice usually appears when a full-term baby is 2 or 3 days old and disappears when she is 4 or 5 days old, although it may last as long as six weeks in breast-fed babies. Jaundice appears in premature babies when they are 3 to 4 days old and disappears when they are 7 to 9 days old. Jaundice that is already present at birth or that appears after the age of one week likely has some other cause and needs to be investigated. All cases of jaundice need to be watched very carefully by the doctor.

Hiccupping and Sneezing Frequent hiccupping and sneezing are normal in newborns and do not usually indicate disease.

Sleeping Newborns sleep much of the time—up to 17 hours a day and as much as four and a half hours at a stretch. Sleeping arrangements are up to you. Some parents and babies disturb each other when they sleep in the same room. For other families, the family bed shared by everyone is preferred.

Spitting Up Lots of healthy babies spit up, many as long as the whole of the first year. Although it sometimes seems that more is coming back up than is being kept down, remember that, when it's spread all over the baby's bib and clothes, it looks like more than it actually is. Rarely does a baby spit up so much that he fails to thrive and grow. Projectile vomiting, though, is something to worry about and to report to the doctor. That's when milk actually shoots like a rocket from the baby's mouth. Green vomit should also be reported to the doctor. It indicates upper gastrointestinal obstruction.

Startling Startling is a normal neurological reflex, described earlier in this chapter in the neurological examination under "Moro Reflex." Although all babies startle, some carry it to extremes. Babies have been known to startle at noises and also in response to being burped or handled. Some even startle when there is no observable cause. As the baby becomes more mature, the neurological system matures, too, and the automatic startle reflex disappears at about 6 months of age.

Urination Baby boys urinate reflexively when exposed to air at diaper-changing time or to warm water at bath time. Observe his urinary stream for the first few weeks of life to be sure that it remains strong. For reasons that are not known, urinary tract infections are three times more common in newborn boys than in girls. One sign of infection is an altered, weakened urinary stream.

NEXT EXAMINATION

Your baby's first well baby checkup will be when she is 2 to 4 weeks old. The visit may be scheduled even sooner if the baby is adopted, had a low birthweight, is jaundiced, or has some other problem the doctor would like to check out.

There are questions the doctor is almost certain to ask you at the first checkup, and it will help if you know about them and are prepared to answer them.

Does the baby seem to see? You can judge your baby's vision by whether or not she seems to look straight into your eyes when you talk to her. You will only be able to hold her attention for brief periods at first, but her attention span will increase rapidly as she grows older. Newborns are also able to turn their eyes toward sounds they hear. If you place an object such as a rattle directly in her line of vision, she may be able to follow it briefly as you move it to midline, the point directly over her nose.

Does the baby seem to hear? Most newborns startle when they hear loud noises. Other responses they make to noise are that they become still for a moment, or their eyes widen.

What about sleeping, eating, and bowel movements? The doctor will probably ask about the baby's sleeping, eating, and bowel movements, so be prepared to report on a typical day.

How are things? Most important, the doctor will probably ask "How are things?" That means how are things with you, the new parents, as well as how are things with the baby. Since the baby's wellbeing is closely linked to your own, it's important that you feel confident, reasonably rested, and physically well. At the same time, it's natural that you feel fatigued sometimes, and you may also be feeling a bit overwhelmed and not a little bit trapped. No matter where you go from now on, the responsibility for your baby goes with you like an invisible umbilical cord that never gets cut. This is a natural feeling.

It's also natural not to be positive all the time about the joys of parenthood. Although most of the time your baby is probably a delight to you, it is also true that babies cry and fuss and soil their diapers and take up a lot of time. It's okay to feel angry and frustrated at least some of the time. If you find yourself feeling that way most of the time, though, or if you think your baby seems to cause you more trouble than other people's babies, mention your feelings to the doctor as soon as possible.

And now a word about friendly advice from a grandmother (or best friend, or sister, or mother-in-law). Don't take it. Listen politely to all the people who offer you surefire advice on childrearing and the latest in homespun medicine if you want to, but remember that this baby is yours. Your own instincts on childraising are probably excellent. As for the baby's health care, that's exclusively the job of the doctor you've chosen for her.

CALLING THE DOCTOR

Call your doctor *before* the next scheduled checkup if your baby has a problem you don't know how to solve, and remember that you may not always talk to the doctor, because a nurse or assistant may be trained to handle certain phone calls. Whether it's after hours or during the day, the doctor would prefer to hear from you only in case of true emergency. She knows, though, that all new parents are anxious, so you'll be forgiven in the beginning for telephoning to report perfectly normal events. But only in the beginning. Here are some tips to help both you and the doctor communicate by telephone.

When to Call Telephone immediately, day or night, in case of the following:
- Loss of consciousness
- Convulsions (body stiffens, eyes deviate to one side, extremities may twitch)
- Breathing difficulties (grunting sounds, ribs showing with breathing, body turning blue)
- Bowel movements that are black or bloody
- Severe diarrhea (three or four episodes of loose, watery stools)

- Rectal temperature of over 101–102°
- Projectile vomiting (shoots into the air) or green vomit
- Unusual crying (baby makes sounds that are different from what you've heard before and that seem abnormal)
- Bloody urine
- No urine for 24 hours

How to call Before you dial, be prepared. Take a pen or pencil and paper to the telephone so you can write down any instructions the doctor or nurse gives you. Have the telephone number of your pharmacy ready to give the doctor in case she wants to phone in a prescription. Explain your baby's problems as accurately as possible. If you're reporting diarrhea or other abnormal bowel movements, for example, describe them and say how long they've been going on and how many episodes there have been.

RESOURCES

American Red Cross Your local Red Cross chapter offers free courses on newborn care and home nursing skills.

Association for Childhood Education International provides pamphlets and booklets on nutrition, education, child care and the family, preschools, and day care. For their publications list, write them at 3615 Wisconsin Avenue N.W., Washington, D.C. 20016.

Community College Education Programs Courses and programs for parent, infant, toddler, and preschool education are offered by your local community colleges and vocational/technical institutions. Call the schools directly for further information.

Consumer Information Index A number of free or low-cost government publications on child care and family concerns are listed in the *Consumer Information Index.* For your free copy, write Public Documents Distribution Center, Pueblo, Colorado 81009.

County Family Services Across the United States

there are county family services associated with United Way and partially funded by them. Call your county or United Way office for the family services nearest you, including family and marriage counseling, parenting classes, and counseling on child abuse. Fees are on a sliding scale according to income.

County Visiting Nurse Service   Local county health departments provide home nurse services as well as homemakers who can help out after the birth of a baby. There are fees for both services, depending on your ability to pay. Homemakers help with household tasks and provide supervision of older children in the family but do not provide care for mother or baby.

La Leche League (LLL)   La Leche League is an international organization of breast-feeding mothers that offers counseling, monthly meetings, and printed information at low cost. For information about the LLL nearest you, write La Leche League International, Inc., 9616 Minneapolis Avenue, Franklin Park, Illinois 60131, or telephone 1-312-455-7730 from 9 A.M. to 3 P.M. Monday through Friday. After 3 P.M. a recorded message refers the caller to a league mother who can answer breast-feeding questions.

National Organization of Mothers of Twins Clubs,   5402 Amberwood Lane, Rockville, Maryland 20853, is a national information services and support group for parents of twins. They can help you find your local group if one exists.

Parents of Prematures (POP)   This group is dedicated to providing emotional and educational support to the parents of preterm or critically ill babies. POP is not yet a national organization, but it exists in most major population areas. To find out if your area has a POP, call the intensive care unit of a local hospital nursery or local childbirth educator organization.

United Way   United Way can provide information on literally hundreds of social and health service agencies available in your area. Call the United Way Community Information Line for further information.

3
SAFETY

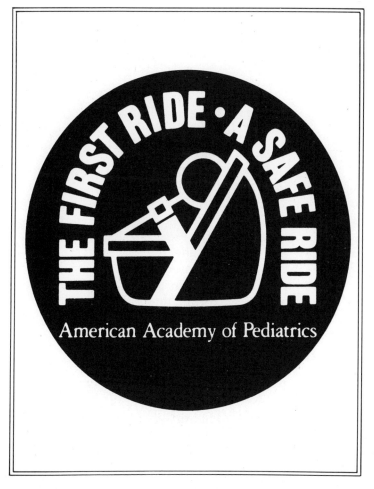

Symbol of the American Academy of Pediatrics'
The First Ride—A Safe Ride program, promoting
crash-tested car seats for infants and children.

It's really hard to talk about safety without sounding preachy, but the safe environment you provide for your baby is one of the most important factors in his getting a good, healthy start in life. Just think of how much effort and skill went into bringing him into the world and taking care of him in the first few critical hours of life. Now the rest is all up to you. After a baby survives the trauma of birth and the first days of life, the greatest threats to his wellbeing are accidents at home (falls, choking, drowning, poisoning, and burns) and in cars. Especially in cars. Auto accidents kill and injure more children each year than anything else, including childhood diseases. So important are safety issues that your baby's doctor will probably talk to you about them at every single checkup from birth through age 2 years and well beyond. We hope this chapter will help you understand why safety is so important to you and your new baby.

BIRTH–4 MONTHS

Equipment   Your first opportunity to protect your newborn comes when you take him home from the hospital. The safest place for your baby is in your arms, right? Wrong. Not when you're both in a moving vehicle. You need a properly installed, crash-tested car seat. Bought, borrowed, or leased (more about that later), it's the most important piece of equipment you'll ever acquire.

Car Seats   The most dangerous place for a baby to be in a car is in your arms. If you were wearing a seat belt, the force of even a low-speed crash would propel him from your grasp headfirst, as if he weighed hundreds of pounds. You couldn't possibly hold on to him. At 30 miles an hour, a 10-pound baby exerts a 300-pound force on impact. An adult becomes a one- or two-ton force. That means that if you were not wearing a seat belt, you would both be thrown forward, and you would severely crush your baby on impact. Or, if you and the baby were both strapped into the same seat belt, your increased weight during a crash would cause the belt to cut deeply into his body.

Next worse is having your newborn strapped into an adult seat belt. Designed for grownups, it would injure his delicate abdomen or hips in case of a crash because he would bear the full force in a single place on his body, where the seat belt was placed. (Note, though, that for older babies—6 to 9 months and more—who can sit up, an adult seat belt is better than no protection at all.) Worse yet is placing a baby, unrestrained, on a passenger seat, particularly in the front of the car.

In short, there's no question about your needing a car seat. But what about choosing it, affording it, and installing it? There are many approved models to choose from. Some can accommodate both infants and toddlers. Others are designed specifically for one or the other. There are also booster seats for youngsters who weigh more than 20 pounds. All have a harness specially designed to distribute the force of a crash over various points on the body. Some are five-point harnesses (shoulders, hips, and crotch), others three-point (shoulders and crotch).

Any car seat that has passed motor vehicle standard 213 is a good choice *provided it can be properly installed in your car.* If, for example, the car seat you choose has a top anchor strap, it *must* be fastened to an anchor plate that has been specially installed in your car. Used without the anchor plate, the seat is much less safe. Your pediatrician or clinic has a list of approved infant seats. One such list is published by the American Academy of Pediatrics (*A Family Shopping Guide To Infant/Child Automobile Restraints,* March 1981). Some clinics even have prescription forms for approved car seats. It is important that you have the most up-to-date information before you make your purchase.

Infant and child car seats range in price from about $25 to $75, with additional costs for special installations. For some families, that is a great deal of money, so it pays to shop around. Prices on the same models often vary from place to place. Some well baby clinics have made special arrangements with retailers to provide car seats at reduced cost. Civic organizations (like the Jaycee Auxiliary), church groups, and insurance companies also offer car seats on loan or for very low fees. Some hospitals, too, have low-cost purchase or rental plans for their patients.

In fact, more and more hospitals, doctors, and communities can be expected to become more involved in car seat programs. So urgent is the issue of car seats and automobile safety that early in 1981 the American Academy of Pediatrics (AAP) launched its The First Ride— A Safe Ride program, a nationwide effort to promote car safety for all infants and children, not only for the first ride but for every ride afterward.

AAP chapters in each state are autonomous in their methods of carrying out the program. In some states legislation has been introduced to make car seats mandatory for children. In several states such laws have already been passed. In others, car safety remains the responsibility of individual doctors and hospitals. One Honolulu obstetrician reported to AAP officials great success with his personal method of enforcing The First Ride—A Safe Ride. During prenatal care and again as he checks mothers-to-be into the hospital, he tells parents that if they have an approved car seat they can take their babies home with them. If not, he will take the baby home. So far, he's never had to take a baby home.

Ideally, it will one day be possible to use car seats in buses, cabs, trains, and other public conveyances, most of which now provide no way to anchor the seats. Meanwhile, it is important for you to have a car seat, *even if you don't have a car,* for those occasions when you and your baby ride in somebody else's car.

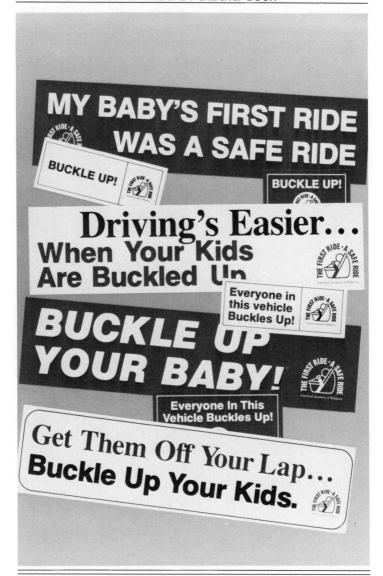

Information on how you can get bumper and dashboard stickers like the ones pictured here is available from your local pediatrician, your local health department, or the American Academy of Pediatrics, P.O. Box 1034, Evanston, Illinois 60204.

Now you know why your pediatrician will ask so many times in the first year whether or not you have an approved car seat for your baby. He'll keep right on asking until he's sure that you have one, that it's approved and properly installed, and that you use it every time you use your automobile.

Never leave your baby unattended in a car. This is a very unsafe practice that can cause serious injury and even death. Cars without drivers have been known to roll and crash; catch fire; and, with windows closed on a hot day, to cause babies and young children to suffocate.

A last word about cars: whatever its political future, the 55-mile-per-hour speed limit has saved thousands of lives on United States highways since it was first imposed as an emergency measure in 1974.

Cribs and Playpens Things you should know about other baby equipment are that the slats on cribs and play-pens should be set no more than 2⅜ inches apart so that babies can't get their heads caught between them. That's a federal law. Mesh playpens must be made of mesh that is fine enough so that a button from a baby's clothing can't become caught in it. The crib mattress should fit snugly and be placed 26 inches below the top of the rails, which should be kept up and in a locked position whenever the baby is in the crib. There should be no decorative cornices or devices at either the head or foot of the crib that could trap the baby's head. There should be no sharp edges anywhere.

Paint, if any, on cribs and all other baby furniture, must be lead-free, for paint that contains lead presents a serious health hazard to babies and young children. Like puppies, they chew on anything—it doesn't have to be food—and if they chew on a lead-painted surface, the result can be lead poisoning.

Lead is a deadly toxin that gets into nerves, bones, and tissue and never comes out. It damages nerves, destroys blood cells, and can cause brain damage and mental retardation when the dose is sufficiently high. Lead poisoning causes severe muscle and nerve pain in affected children, especially in the abdomen. A long series of treatments is required for heavily poisoned children, but damage is usually severe and permanent. Note that in order to be safe, a piece of furniture must never have been painted with lead paint. New coats of safe paint applied over an old coat of lead paint do not erase the danger, for a child can easily chew right down to the toxic layer.

Infant Seats If you buy or borrow an infant seat, remember that it isn't sturdy enough to double as a car seat. Don't leave your baby unattended in it on high places such as kitchen counters or table tops. Newborns can't knock their infant seats over—although by the time they are a few weeks old, they can do so easily—but siblings and inquisitive house pets can. Keep the infant seat on the floor or *tied* to a sturdy chair.

For carrying your baby on outdoor excursions, choose a sling-type front carrier until he is about 4 months old. Until then, he won't have enough head control to be carried in a back carrier. These don't give any support at all to his head.

Equipment that is loaned to you or acquired at a garage sale or second-hand shop is no bargain if it's unsafe. Some models of toys and equipment, *officially recalled by the manufacturer for being dangerous,* are still available in attics and garages and on the second-hand market. Although federal product safety standards do apply to second-hand stores, they are not always rigidly enforced. However you get it, be sure you get good, safe equipment for your baby. If in doubt, call the Consumer Products Safety Commission hotline number—1-800-638-8326. See the resources section at the end of this chapter for details.

Pacifiers Even a pacifier can be lethal if it's not properly constructed. It should be a sturdy, single-piece construction, since multiple parts may separate and be swallowed by the baby. It should not have a long cord attached that could entangle and strangle the baby. And it should be checked periodically to be sure it hasn't been weakened by sterilization or the baby's sucking.

Burns   You may even need to be concerned about the clothes your baby wears. By federal law, baby and child sleepwear must be flameproof. One flame retardant called Tris was banned from the market in 1977 after it was linked to cancer. At that time thousands of pieces of children's sleepwear treated with Tris were recalled and sold as industrial rags. Some of the banned sleepwear, however, was resold and became available to unsuspecting consumers as recently as last year in discount and second-hand stores. Be suspicious of sleepwear that doesn't have its original label and lacks information about the flame retardant used in its manufacture. Labels also provide laundering instructions, which must be followed carefully in order to preserve the flameproof nature of the garment.

An excellent way to prevent your baby's being accidentally scalded is to turn the thermostat on your home water heater down to 52° C (120–130°F). Thin and delicate, a baby's skin scalds easily. It takes just a few seconds of exposure to water at a higher temperature to injure a baby seriously.

Falls   To prevent an accidental fall, keep an eye *and a hand* on your baby at all times. You'll notice that when you bring him in for his checkups, someone will keep a hand on his tummy whenever he's on the examining table. It's a good practice for you, too. Babies begin to roll over at about age 2 months, but some do it as early as 6 weeks, and even a newborn moves himself by pulling his legs up under his body and then straightening them again. When babies roll over, they can fall off chairs, counter tops, and beds with lightning speed. Don't leave your baby on top of anything unless you're there beside him with a firm hold on him.

4–6 MONTHS

Take inventory of your home now for small objects that could accidentally be swallowed by your baby. At age 4 months he can grasp objects in his fist and bring them to his mouth. If they are too small, he may swallow and choke

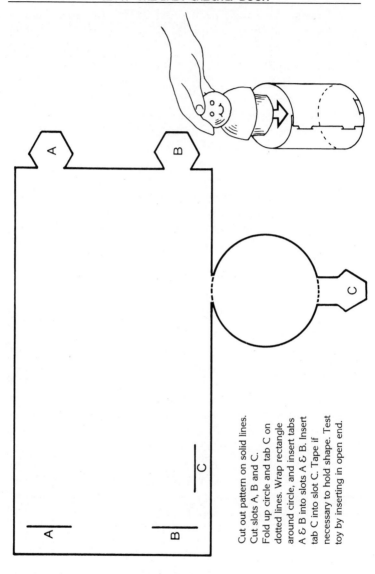

Cut out pattern on solid lines.
Cut slots A, B and C.
Fold up circle and tab C on dotted lines. Wrap rectangle around circle, and insert tabs A & B into slots A & B. Insert tab C into slot C. Tape if necessary to hold shape. Test toy by inserting in open end.

If an object fits through the hole at the top of this cylinder, it is a danger to your baby.

on them. Your baby has a mitten-grasp method for holding things now, but very soon he'll be able to use his thumb and forefinger to pick up, and pick at, small objects like the eyes on his teddy bear. Many stuffed animals have eyes that babies can swallow and choke on. Some eyes are even attached to the animals with two-inch spikes! Now is a good time to remove the eyes on all your baby's stuffed toys and replace them with embroidered eyes.

Other dangerous toys include squeeze toys with whistles that can be picked out and swallowed and all other toys with small parts. In fact, the United States government has addressed itself to the small-parts problem. There are federal safety regulations that protect children younger than 3 years from the danger of swallowing and choking on small parts. The regulations prohibit the manufacture of small toys or removable small parts on toys intended for those children. Toys or parts of toys intended for babies must *not* be able to fit into a cylinder with a diameter of 1¼ inches and a slanted bottom. The cylinder is sized and shaped as closely as possible to the windpipe of a small child. It is legal to produce small-parts toys for youngsters older than age 3 years, however, so your 4-month-old has to be protected from his older brother or sister's toys.

Also dangerous are toys suspended from cords that hang too close to the crib. The best policy with any toy attached to a cord is to cut the cord. There is also danger of accidental strangulation from window-shade and drapery cords when the crib is placed too close to the window.

Equipment

Baby Carriers, Jumpers, and Walkers Baby's head control is good enough now so that he can be carried in a backpack-type baby carrier. His improved head control also means he can use a jumper or a walker, both of which are a real treat for most babies. Construction should be checked for sturdiness and to be sure there are no sharp edges. Jumpers should be constructed with their own base. Those that are suspended from door frames and ceilings are dangerous because they can come loose. Walkers are the subject of some medical controversy. Some doctors believe that they are dangerous, and further, that they disrupt motor development. The danger lies in the high speeds at which babies can propel themselves in a walker. Collisions, falling down stairs, and tipping over doorjambs are three major problems. The most common injuries are cuts, scrapes, and bruises. As for motor development, it has been suggested that babies who spend a lot of time in walkers grow lazy about their creeping and walking skills and may show a delay in them.

Much depends, of course, on your home situation. If you live in a small apartment, there's probably little danger of your baby being able to travel a great enough distance to build up much speed. But if you reside in a roomy house with lots of open space, several levels, and stairs, it's conceivable your baby could build up a pretty good head of steam as he travels from place to place. As for a walker's disrupting development, much depends on the common sense of the parent. If a baby were in the walker most of the time, it might indeed make a difference in his motor skills. So would anything that he was subjected to all day, such as being left howling in his carriage or abandoned in his playpen.

High Chairs Choose a chair with sturdy construction, with a broad base that cannot be tipped over easily. Always be sure the strap that holds the baby is secure and fastened. A separate harness is highly recommended, and there should not only be a restraint around the waist but through the crotch as well.

Babies have a universal trick of stiffening their bodies, arching their backs, and throwing their heads back. They save this trick exclusively for their high chairs, and it causes them to shoot straight out of the chairs feet first, like little torpedoes. Restaurant high chairs can be a problem if the straps are missing or not in working condition. Having your own harness with you means never having to worry about it.

Infant Seat Your baby has pretty much outgrown his infant seat by now. He can tip it over easily. It is recommended that you discontinue its use no later than when your baby reaches 5 months of age.

6 MONTHS

At age 6 months your baby is getting ready. In the weeks and months to come, his ability to creep, stand, climb, walk, and run will all increase remarkably. Along with the increase in his physical prowess comes an increase in danger to your child and an increase in the safety measures you will have to take in order to protect him. Fortunately, there are precautions you can take now to protect your baby from becoming a statistic. The most important are childproofing your home, acquiring a good first aid book, and learning some first aid principles to be used in case of emergency.

Childproofing the House   Take a few minutes to think like a baby and look at things from your baby's point of view. Imagine you are down on all fours, looking at each room in the house from that vantage point. Everything you see is new and wonderful, to be poked, grabbed, handled, sucked, and chewed. You have no sense of danger or hurt. You haven't learned yet to make mental connections between your own actions and the possible consequences. When you pull yourself to stand at a small table, you don't know it can topple over on you. You have no idea that soup in a bowl or coffee in a cup can scald and burn or that an electrical wall outlet can shock, burn, and even kill.

The following suggestions apply to all rooms in your house or apartment.

- Buy safety caps for electric wall outlets. These cost only pennies each and are available in supermarkets, hardware stores, and five-and-dime stores.
- Put rubber mats under scatter rugs that slide out from underfoot.
- Place safety gates at the tops and bottoms of stairs, and keep stairwells well lighted.
- Keep all doors that lead to danger latched or locked—steps to the basement, for example.
- Keep all medicines in containers with childproof caps and stored safely out of reach. Use a locked cabinet if possible.

- Keep small objects that can be swallowed and choked on (buttons, pins, parts of older children's toys) either locked up or out of reach.
- Keep windows locked or screened.
- Check your house plants. Many are poisonous if eaten. Others, though not poisonous, may cause choking if a baby tries to eat them.

POISONOUS HOUSE PLANTS*

Plant	Toxic Part	Symptoms
Asparagus fern	Young shoots	Painful skin inflammation
Castor bean	Seeds	Nausea, vomiting, diarrhea, burning sensation in mouth and throat, possible convulsions and urinary complications
Christmas cherry (see Jerusalem cherry)		
Crown of thorns	Entire plant	Blistering, irritation, rash, severe pain if rubbed in eye
Daffodil	Bulb	Nausea, vomiting, and diarrhea
Devil's ivy (pothos)	All parts	Severe burning and irritation of mouth; base of tongue may swell and block airway
Dieffenbachia	All parts	Same as devil's ivy

*Based on information provided by the Children's Orthopedic Hospital Medical Center (COHMC) Poison Center, Seattle.

POISONOUS HOUSE PLANTS

Plant	Toxic Part	Symptoms
English ivy	All parts	Nausea, vomiting, diarrhea, headache, excitement, breathing difficulty, coma
Hyacinth	Bulb	Nausea, vomiting, diarrhea
Jerusalem cherry (also called Christmas cherry)	Leaves and fruit, especially unripe fruit	Severe stomach pain, vomiting, diarrhea, headache, circulatory and respiratory depression, shock
Oleander	All parts	Severe digestive upset; also affects heart
Mistletoe	All parts	Mild intestinal irritation and diarrhea
Narcissus	Bulb	Nausea, vomiting, diarrhea
Philodendron	All parts	Severe burning and irritation of mouth and tongue; base of tongue may swell and block airway
Poinsettia	Leaves	Not as toxic as previously thought
Rosary pea	Seeds	Nausea, vomiting, diarrhea, burning sensation in mouth and throat, possible convulsions and urinary complications

The plants listed here are only a few of the poisonous ones with which a child might come in contact. Others include ornamental shrubs like azaleas, sometimes brought indoors before planting, or vegetable plants like tomatoes, occasionally started up indoors before being transferred to the garden. When your child is older and begins to play out of doors, the danger from poisonous plants increases greatly. Dozens of plants found in flower and vegetable gardens are toxic, as are many trees, shrubs, and wild plants.

For safety's sake, keep labels on all your house plants. If you see your child eating a plant, call your poison center or doctor to determine whether or not it is poisonous and to get instructions on what to do. If you take your child to the doctor's office or a hospital emergency room, take a large clipping of the plant with you, including leaves and berries, if any. And remember that even if a plant isn't poisonous, a child who tries to eat it may choke on it.

Kitchen
- Check to be sure the handles on pots and pans don't extend over the stove top as a temptation for baby to grab.
- Use the back burners for cooking whenever possible when baby is present.
- Don't keep anything on counter tops within reach of baby.
- Keep baby's high chair away from stove, counter tops, and baseboard heaters.
- Keep electric appliance cords away from baby's reach.
- Keep knives and scissors out of reach.
- Don't leave baby unsupervised near a table set with tablecloth or placemats that can be pulled off, dumping glassware or hot food on baby.
- Move bleaches, cleaning agents, and detergents to a high shelf.
- Give baby a drawer or cupboard of his own, filled with things that are okay and safe for him to play

with, like rolling pins, pots and pot lids, and measuring cups.
• Move kitchen poisons out of reach to a high shelf. These include ammonia, bleach, detergents, disinfectants, furniture polish and wax, insecticides, lighter fluid, lye and drain cleaners, oven cleaners, shoe dye and polish, and many other substances.

Living Room
• Remove knickknacks and other objects small enough to be swallowed.
• Keep lamp cords out of reach. Tape them to the underside of tables and down the backside of table legs. When babies chew on electric cords, their mouths may be severely burned. It's a common injury.
• Remove heavy or sharp objects from coffee and occasional tables.
• Be sure second-hand furniture has been painted with lead-free paint.
• Keep cigarettes, matches, and lighters out of reach.
• Keep a basket or other container full of things that are safe and okay for baby to play with.
• Living room poisons are mostly associated with house plants. See pages 66-67.

Bathroom
• Keep drugs, soaps, and sprays out of reach. Drugs should be stored in containers with childproof caps in a locked medicine cabinet if possible.
• Keep razor blades out of reach.
• Don't leave baby unattended in bathtub even for a few seconds.
• Bathroom poisons include all medications, such as aspirin, vitamins, and iron. Also poisonous are lotions, linaments, salves, and toilet bowl cleaners.

Baby's Room
• NO SMOKING.
• Lead-free paint on all furniture.

- Keep crib away from windows, heaters, and shade/drapery window cords.
- Keep crib sides locked in up position.

Parents' Bedroom
- Plants may be poisonous. Check the poison plant chart.
- Bedroom poisons include deodorants, hair sprays and conditioners, mothballs, nail polish and remover.

First Aid   After you've childproofed the house, it's time to think about first aid. Buy a good first aid book. See "Resources" at the end of this chapter for recommendations. It's not enough to have a first aid book in the house, though. You have to read it and familiarize yourself with basic first aid principles. The more you know, the better able you'll be to help another family member in an emergency until professional help arrives.

A knowledge of mouth-to-mouth resuscitation and cardiopulmonary resuscitation (CPR) are indispensable. Fortunately, they're not hard to learn. In fact, children age 12 and up learn both techniques easily. Mouth-to-mouth resuscitation involves pinching the nose and breathing into the mouth of a person who has stopped breathing (after you're sure the mouth and throat are clear). CPR combines mouth-to-mouth with manual chest compressions to provide breathing *and* blood flow for a person who not only has stopped breathing but whose heart has stopped as well. These are simple techniques and proven lifesavers. They are vital for all parents and older children to know about. See "Resources" at the end of this chapter for information on the availability of CPR courses.

The following information about the most common injuries to children—falls, inhalation of foreign objects, drowning, poisoning, and burns—is not meant to be a substitute for a first aid book and professional help, for there is none. It merely outlines some principles about the injuries themselves.

Falls   Often with babies and young children, falls are headfirst from heights. Any suspicion of head injury should be reported to your doctor, who will probably want to check to see that the baby's pupils are working correctly and that his level of consciousness is normal. As for injured extremities, it's pretty hard for a parent to examine a pudgy little arm or leg for abnormal swelling, but there are other indications of injury. After a fall, the baby may begin to favor an extremity or stop using it entirely. This is fairly easy to notice, since all of a baby's movements are normally symmetrical. If you see that the baby is favoring a limb or not using it at all, you should call the doctor immediately.

Inhalation (Aspiration) of Foreign Objects   You already know that babies put everything possible into their mouths, so there's a real danger of their aspirating (inhaling and choking on) small objects. If you wait for help when your baby is choking, that help could come too late. It's up to you to know how to force the swallowed object out of the child's windpipe.

Drowning   A victim of near-drowning requires immediate mouth-to mouth resuscitation or cardiopulmonary resuscitation (CPR) at the site of the accident *plus* special followup care and evaluation in a hospital.

An enjoyable way of helping to prevent water accidents is to take family swimming lessons with your baby. Parent-taught courses are available in both private and public pools in your community. Although early experience with water helps babies to develop preswimming skills such as breath holding, blowing bubbles, and endurance, age 3 years is considered by some to be the earliest age appropriate for actual swimming lessons. And whether or not your baby has had preswimming lessons, he must be carefully watched whenever he is near water. The Council on Child and Adolescent Health of the American Academy of Pediatrics cautions that no young child can ever be considered "water safe" and that any swimming program should be on a one-to-one basis with the parent or a responsible adult. They suggest, further, that babies with medical problems should have clearance first from their doctors.

Information on swimming lessons is available from your local chapter of the American Red Cross. They do not accept youngsters less than 3 years old, but they can make recommendations.

Poisoning   A number of poisons, including poisonous plants, are mentioned in this chapter, but the list is far from complete. Remember that *any* substance that isn't food can be poisonous when eaten by a baby or small child and should be reported to a poison center or doctor. Don't wait for symptoms. Call.

Never do anything to or for a poison victim without specific instructions from a poison-control center or doctor. Some poisons, like dishwasher detergent and lye, are caustic. That is, they quickly burn whatever they touch. Vomiting should never be induced for this kind of poisoning because the vomited material injures a second time everything with which it comes in contact. Caustic poisons also burn the mouths of rescuers who attempt to resuscitate the victim. With other kinds of poisons, the victim should be forced to vomit. Syrup of ipecac, available without prescription at all pharmacies, is a preparation that induces vomiting. Your baby's doctor will suggest that you buy some for an emergency. *However, you should never give it to your child unless you have been instructed to do so by the poison-control center or your doctor.*

Families are at risk for accidental poisoning when there is a disruption in the usual routine—when a family member is sick, grandparents are visiting, or the family is moving, for example. Accidental poisonings are also more likely to occur in younger children during the hubbub and distraction of getting older children off to school or, in the evening, of getting everybody off to bed. Prevention is, of course, the best defense against poisoning. Keep syrup of ipecac on hand, and have the grandparents buy some, too. Keep the poison center phone number by the phone, and attach Mr. Yuk stickers to anything that's poisonous. Mr. Yuk was developed by the Children's Hospital of Pittsburgh and has been adopted by many poison-control centers

*Mr. Yuk, the poison warning symbol of the
National Poison Center Network, Children's
Hospital of Pittsburgh. Reprinted by permission.*

throughout the country. Free stickers are available at your
local center, also at pharmacies.

Most important, keep all medications in a safe place.
And never tell a child that medicine is candy.

Burns   Burns, even minor ones, should be evaluated
by a doctor as soon as possible. Untreated and allowed to
become infected, even a first-degree burn can be serious.
Burns of the hands and feet, no matter how superficial they
appear, can scar, for a baby's skin is thinner and more
sensitive than a grownup's. It burns much more easily and
suffers far more damage. All major burns should be treated
in a special burn center. Butter or greasy ointments should
not be applied to burns. Burns should not be sprayed with
pain-killing agents. A cool, clean, wet cloth may be applied
to the injured area as a first aid measure. Remember that a
burn can be caused by three sources—heat, chemicals,
and electricity. A good safety measure is to lower the
temperature on your home water heater.

ONE YEAR

The chase is on. The one-year-old walks—by herself, holding on to someone's hand, or cruising sideways along furniture. Her curiosity is greater than her common sense. Very simply, she needs to be watched but not curtailed. If you haven't thoroughly childproofed your home, bought a first aid book, and mastered some basic first aid principles, now is definitely the time to do so.

Remember that the greatest threats to a baby in the first year of life are falls, burns, choking, drowning, poisoning, and automobile accidents.

2 YEARS

Without your help and supervision, a 2-year-old child is an accident waiting to happen. Many months ago (we hope) you childproofed your home to protect her from falls, burns, electric shocks, and accidental poisonings. Now you need to extend your concern for her safety to the backyard, street, and neighborhood. The ideal yard is fenced with childproof locks at the entrance. Even so, a 2-year-old always needs supervision when playing outdoors. She also needs to be taught that the street means danger and that she should never step into it unless an adult is holding her hand.

Be sure that any play equipment in your yard has been properly assembled and installed. It should be placed away from fences and walls and there should be a safe surface underneath, such as sand or sawdust. Climbing gyms, swings, slides, and seesaws should never be placed over surfaces such as cement, aggregate, asphalt, or gravel. Check the equipment periodically for damage and make repairs promptly.

There are voluntary safety standards for all the playground equipment manufactured in the United States. The resulting designs are supposed to be safe and free from rough and sharp edges and other safety hazards. But even though the equipment may be well designed and properly installed and maintained, you will still need to train your youngster in its safe use. Slides are for feet-first, not head-first use, for example. Jungle gyms and monkey bars are for hanging on, not for tightrope walking. In any case, a 2-year-old is not old enough to use any piece of playground equipment without supervision.

RESOURCES

The U.S. Consumer Product Safety Commission (CPSC) is an independent regulatory agency charged with reducing the risk of injury associated with consumer products. *Toll-free hotline numbers:* 1-800-638-8326 or 1-800-638-8333. In Maryland: 1-800-492-8363. The hotline answers from 8:30 A.M. to 6 P.M., Eastern time. During nonworking hours, messages are recorded and answered on the following work day. The CPSC cannot make recommendations or give advice on the phone, but it will give information on a specific product you have questions about. So know the manufacturer, model, and serial number of the product about whose safety you're concerned.

The CPSC has a list of recalled and banned toys and children's equipment, which they will send on request. They also have a number of publications, available free, on childhood safety, children's furniture, playground equipment, poisons, and toys. Write for the free *Catalogue of Publications,* U.S. Consumer Product Safety Commission, Washington, D.C., 20207.

The CPSC has regional and district offices in Atlanta, Boston, Chicago, Twin Cities, Cleveland, Dallas, Kansas City, Denver, Los Angeles, New York, Philadelphia, San Francisco, and Seattle.

First Aid Books

A Sigh of Relief. Martin I. Green. New York: Bantam Books, 1977. ($6.95) Well illustrated and written, this book is all about childhood emergencies and written so that a child of 10 or so could conceivably use it to help a younger child in distress. A single criticism is that cardiopulmonary resuscitation (CPR) is not identified as such, although the procedure does appear under the heading "Heart Failure."

Standard First Aid and Personal Safety. The American National Red Cross. Garden City: Doubleday & Co., Inc., 1979. This is a classic—easy to read, well illustrated, and available for only $2.50 from your local Red Cross chapter.

Cardiopulmonary Resuscitation (CPR)

Information about instruction is available from your local hospital, police station, fire station, or the local chapters of the American Heart Association and American Red Cross. It is also available through adult education and school programs in your community.

Parent-Taught Preswimming Lessons   Information is available from your local YMCA, Red Cross, city/county pools, and private pool owners.

4
THE
PHYSICAL
EXAMINATION

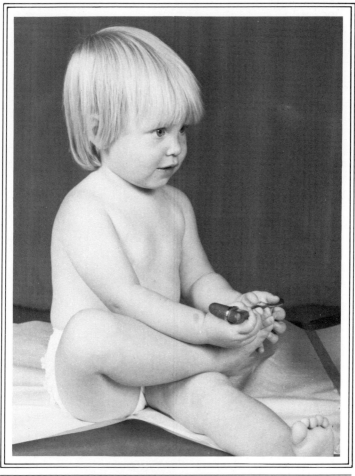

✓ CHECKLIST

STANDARD PHYSICAL EXAMINATION

_____ Head
_____ Neck
_____ Arms and underarms
_____ Hands
_____ Abdomen
_____ Legs
_____ Feet
_____ Hips
_____ Femoral pulses in the groin
_____ Genitals
_____ Back and Spine
_____ Anus

WITH INSTRUMENTS

_____ Heart
_____ Lungs
_____ Eyes
_____ Nose
_____ Mouth and throat
_____ Ears

In the first two years of his life a child has more routine physical examinations than he will ever have again in so short a period of time. The physical examination is a key part of every well baby checkup. It can yield important information about each system in the developing child—the brain and nervous system, the musculoskeletal system (muscle and bone development), the cardiovascular system (heart and lungs), and, to some extent, even how the child is developing socially. This is done by observing the child's behavior during the exam as well as his interactions with his parents. The exam is also used to monitor partially the acuteness of vision and hearing. True diagnostic tests for good vision and hearing cannot be performed until the child is older, however.

In addition to checking up on how a child is developing mentally, physically, and socially, the physical examination serves as a screening device for disease. It can uncover conditions such as ear and urinary-tract infections that may have gone unnoticed because the child showed no symptoms, but that left untreated, could eventually cause serious complications, such as hearing loss and kidney disease.

Even though a complete physical examination isn't mandatory at every single well baby checkup, many doctors choose to perform the exam each time because it can yield so much important information and because it takes so little time. A skilled examiner can perform a complete examination in a matter of a few minutes. For most doctors, then, there's no reason *not* to do a complete physical examination at each well baby checkup. Later, though, when your child is older, he may become balky, frightened, and uncooperative during some parts of the examination. In that case, the doctor may skip a step or two in the examination process, but only if he believes the child to be in excellent general health. Remember that every doctor has a different style and a different order of doing things. The maneuvers described in this chapter may not always be performed, because the doctor modifies the exam based on what he knows about your child.

When the doctor enters the examining room, says hello, and begins to wash his hands, he has already begun the examination. He is observing the baby's general appearance and how comfortable you are with your child. He is noticing the baby's level of activity, his alertness, and how he reacts to his surroundings. If you brought more than one child to the checkup, the doctor is able to observe sibling (brother/sister) relationships as well.

Many doctors begin by asking, "How are things?" This gives parents an opportunity right away to mention any problems they are having. The question is meant to uncover problems, and you should feel free to answer it honestly. In our society when friends meet and say, "How are you?" they don't really want to know. But in this case the doctor really does want to know, so you should be prepared to mention all of your concerns during the course of the checkup. The doctor may respond by wanting to discuss a concern immediately or by suggesting that it be postponed until the end of the examination, when there is still another opportunity for talk between doctor and parent.

After the "How are things?" doctors often ask questions concerning previous problems to make sure they've been resolved. Questions like "Does he still seem to be having a problem with his ears?" or "Has his sister gotten used to having him around yet?" are usual at this point in the exam. Take this as an opportunity. Be completely honest when you answer questions because that's the only way the doctor can really help.

For most families, raising children is a positive, happy experience. But it is also a complex, challenging, and long-term event, and *everybody* needs help with it at one time or another. It's okay to need help. There is no problem you could possibly share with the doctor that would shock him, and he is not there to make moral judgments, either. If there are family problems, he can either help directly or refer you to other professionals who can. It's all part of his job as your baby's doctor. Problems within the family are sure to have some effect on the child's wellbeing, so they are an integral part of the doctor's concern. Whether he is a pediatrician, a general practitioner, or a specialist in family practice, the doctor will try to keep the whole family in mind when treating the child.

Before "laying hands" on the baby, the doctor will finish his visual observations, noting if there are any rashes or other skin lesions and whether the skin is flushed, pale, or normal in color. He looks for equal range of motion and equal vigor on both sides of the baby's body when she kicks with her legs and waves her arms. He talks to the baby and evaluates whether or not she seems to attend (pay attention) to him.

A complete physical examination is a head-to-toe check that includes about a baker's dozen maneuvers. They are not always performed in the same order—in fact, much depends on the child's mood and level of cooperation—but generally the doctor starts with procedures that are least disturbing and frightening (examining the hands by holding them in his own) and works up to the things that most children hate (examination of the ears with the otoscope). Medically, that's known as starting peripherally and working centrally. Translated, that means "Do whatever you can get away with, and do it fast."

Head The doctor runs his fingers over the baby's head, feeling for bulges or lopsidedness. These might indicate that the sutures, the open spaces between the bony

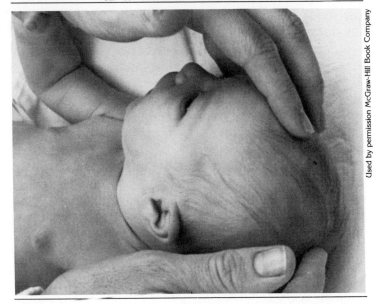

Used by permission McGraw-Hill Book Company

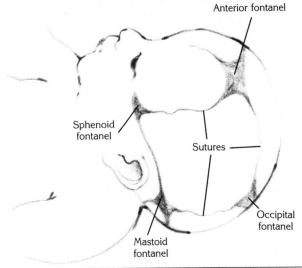

Anterior fontanel

Sphenoid
fontanel

Sutures

Occipital
fontanel

Mastoid
fontanel

*The top of the head is carefully felt for shape
and any abnormal fusion of the sutures. Special
attention is given to examination of the anterior fontanel
to determine the size and to detect any tendency for the
tissues inside the skull to bulge outward.*

plates in the child's head, have joined together, or fused, too early and that the fast-growing brain is being restrained. This in turn would cause the head to grow in an odd, asymmetrical shape.

The doctor also checks the anterior fontanel, the soft spot on top of the baby's head. This spot can get bigger after birth, but it usually begins to get small at about age 6 months and can close anywhere from age 9 to 18 months. When it disappears for good, it means that the skull has fused permanently at the top of the head. As you can see from the drawing at the left, there are actually six fontanels on the baby's head, although it is the top one that gets the most attention and is usually the last to close. All the fontanels represent areas where the brain has been given growing room.

Checking for head control is another important part of the examination for the first six months. At each checkup the doctor lifts the baby from the examining table by both arms to see how much head control he has, how much his head lags behind his body as he is raised from a lying-down position. Newborns have little head control. Their heads sag as they are lifted. At 2 to 3 months, babies have somewhat improved head control and are able to support their own heads slightly as they are raised to sit. The 4-month-old has pretty good control of his head and shows little or no head lag. He brings his head up in a straight line with his body as he is pulled to sit. The 6-month-old has complete head control. Not only does he hold his head erect easily, but his head actually leads his body in anticipation as he is pulled to sit. Head control is the first order of business for a baby, whose development begins with the head and then proceeds in an orderly way to the trunk/body and extremities—arms, legs, hands, and feet.

Neck   The neck is examined primarily for lymph nodes and range of motion. Lymph nodes are pea-sized collections of lymphocytes, the special white cells responsible for the body's immune system. There are five sets of lymph nodes located in the neck and just above the collarbone. Normally nodes are tiny and can't be felt. When they

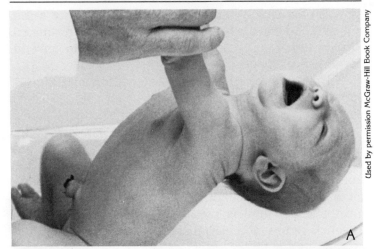

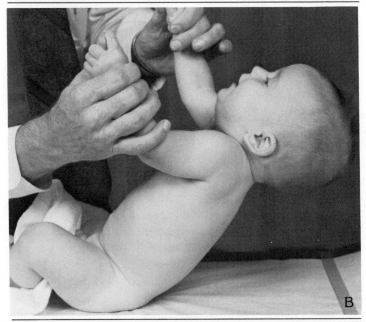

Used by permission McGraw-Hill Book Company

Newborns have very little head control; their heads fall backward when they are lifted (A). By 4 months, babies are able to support their own heads, though the head may still lag a bit behind (B).

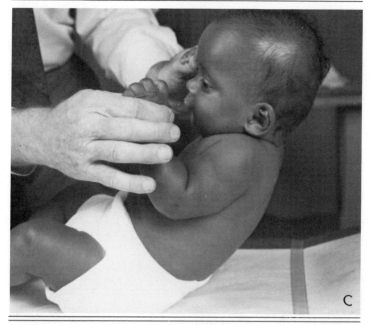

The 6-month-old has complete control;
the head actually leads the body when the child is raised
to a sitting position (C).

become big and hard and you can feel them, it is a sign of illness or infection.

The examiner may turn the baby's head from one side to the other, checking the range of motion and the amount of resistance to movement. Normally the child should be able to turn his head so that his chin reaches the level of his shoulder on each side.

The thyroid gland in the neck is also checked for enlargement (goiter) and for masses. Finally, the trachea (windpipe) is felt. With his fingers the doctor can detect any abnormal tug that would indicate a heart abnormality.

Arms and Underarms The underarms are checked for enlargement or hardening of lymph nodes located there. The arms are checked for mobility and for any swell-

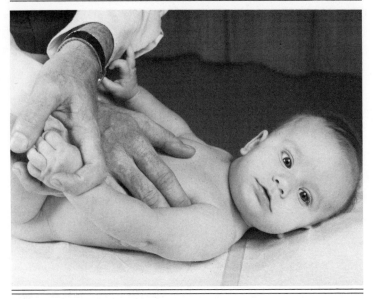

*The underarms are felt to detect enlargement
of the lymph nodes located there.*

ing or tenderness of the joints. Sometimes the reflexes
located near the elbow are tested with a rubber hammer.

Hands Examination of the hands is a nonthreaten-
ing procedure and therefore the one that some doctors
choose to begin with when a young patient is anxious. The
doctor examines the fingers, fingernails, and joints. The
fingers may provide a clue to the abnormal functioning of
the pulmonary (lung) system. See "The Lungs," following.
With an infant, the doctor may also place his finger or other
object in the baby's hand to check the grasp reflex.

Abdomen For the purpose of thorough examination, the belly area is divided into four quarters (quadrants),
and each sector is palpated (felt) carefully for abnormal
masses and enlarged internal organs. Sometimes the doctor has to push quite deeply into the stomach during the
exam. He watches the child's face carefully for any change
of facial expression that would indicate discomfort or pain.

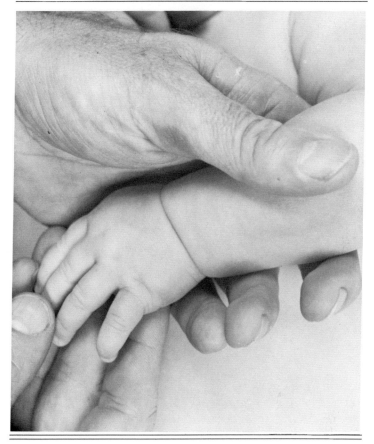

*Hands are examined for color of the
skin and nail beds and any malformations.*

Normally there is no pain. In fact, ticklishness is more often
the problem with young children. Usually the liver can be
felt in the upper right quadrant. Sometimes the tip of the
spleen can be felt there as well. The doctor can also listen to
bowel sounds by placing the stethoscope on the stomach.
The instrument picks up the gurgling sounds of a healthy
intestinal tract.

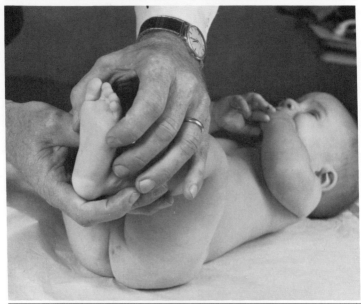

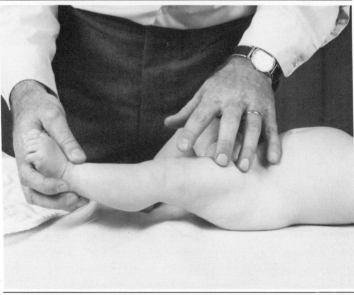

*Feet and legs are examined for malformations.
The legs are stretched out to determine
whether they are straight and can move freely.*

Legs   The legs are stretched out together and observed for straightness and sameness in length. Although many newborns and toddlers appear to be bow-legged, it is something of an optical illusion. Stretching the legs out, the doctor draws an imaginary line starting at the hipbone (the iliac crest) and moving downward through the bump under the kneecap (the tibial tuberosity) and on to the middle toe. If the line is straight, so is the child's leg. Legs are also checked for range of motion to see that both are equal. Joints are checked for swelling or tenderness, and sometimes the patellar (knee-jerk) reflex is tested with a rubber hammer.

Feet   By looking at the foot from the sole, the doctor can see if it's in a normal position at rest. If there is an exaggerated curve on the inside edge of the foot, it indicates toeing-in (metatarsus varus). The outside edge of the foot should be straight.

For about the first two years of life, the feet look quite flat. This is because of a fat pad located under the metatarsal arch. The pad gradually disappears as the baby grows older.

Femoral Pulses in the Groin   An important part of every examination for at least the first year is to feel the pulses located on either side of the groin. These pulses are the primary indication of the quality of blood flow from the aorta of the heart. An equally strong, steady beat on both sides is normal.

Hips   Examination of the hips is one of the most important maneuvers in the physical examination and may be performed at every checkup through age 2 years. In the beginning, babies don't have very well-formed hip sockets, so it is crucial to check them frequently to be sure they are developing normally. With the baby on her back, the doctor draws both her knees up toward her chest and then spreads them apart, froglike, until they touch the examining table. This is called abducting the hips. As the hips are moved, the doctor can feel a click that would indicate that the top of the hipbone (femur) has slipped out of the hip socket (acetabulum). Slipping is abnormal. If the hip can be displaced

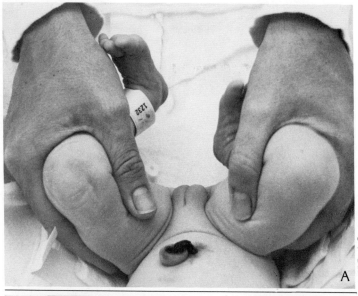

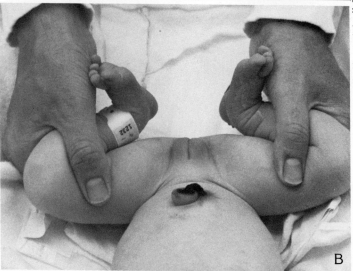

Examination of the hips is very important. The legs are drawn up (A) and then into a froglike position (B) while the doctor feels over the hip joint to detect any tendency for the hip to slip out of its socket.

during the examination, it means the child will surely displace it regularly when she becomes active and begins to creep, walk, and climb.

The danger with displaced hips is that the major blood vessel at the top of the femur can be damaged eventually as the hipbone slips in and out. If blood supply to the hip is cut off, the hipbone is effectively ruined, with arthritis of the hip the usual outcome. Congenitally displaced hips can easily be corrected, but it is important to diagnose and treat them early for best results.

For most babies, hip abduction is not a bothersome procedure. Others, though, have "tight" hips with a slightly restricted range of motion. For them the procedure is a bit uncomfortable, and they are likely to complain about it. Tight hips are not a sign of dislocation, particularly if the tightness is the same on both sides.

Genitals (Genitalia) Boys' genitals are observed for foreskin problems, undescended testicles, and hygiene. The genitals of girls are examined for normal external development and hygiene.

For the first one to three years, the foreskin of an uncircumcised male may not retract easily and should not be forced. Normal bathing will keep the tip of the penis sufficiently clean. The doctor checks the position of the urethral meatus—the opening through which the child urinates. He also feels to see if the testicles are present, as they should be, and that there are no abnormal masses such as hernias.

Hernias in boys often show up as a swelling of the scrotum, the sac that holds the testicles. The swelling is caused by slippage of abdominal tissues into the scrotum. Since hernias slide in and out quite freely, it may be necessary to make the child cry to detect the swelling. His crying forces the hernia into the scrotum, where the doctor can feel it.

The genitals of girls are checked for the normal development of the outer structures—the skin folds called the labia—the opening of the vagina, and the urethra, through which the baby urinates. Hygiene is especially important. If the genitals are not carefully cleaned between the folds, contaminated material can easily collect there and cause infection.

Back and Spine A baby's back is examined as she lies on her stomach, while toddlers sit or stand for this part of the examination. The doctor runs his fingers lightly up and down the length of the spine, or backbone, checking for abnormal bumps that might indicate a spinal defect. During the first six months, the position of the spine and straightness of the back are noted as the baby is pulled to a sitting position. In the early months, the back and spine are normally curved and rounded as the baby leans forward in a sitting position. They straighten markedly at about 6 months of age, when the baby is able to sit by herself without help. Older children (3 years or more) are asked to

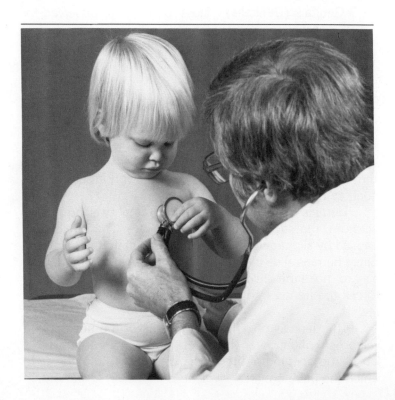

bend down and touch their toes, a movement that reveals abnormal curvature of the spine.

Anus Spreading the buttocks apart, the examiner makes a quick check of the anus. He is looking for fissures and, rarely, fistulas. Fissures are small slits or cracks around the anus that are painful for the baby. They indicate a problem with bowel movements. When movements are too big or too hard, they can create fissures, which can also be caused by overbrisk cleaning of the baby's sensitive bottom. Fistulas are painful swellings with discharge, the remnants of an anal abscess. They usually require surgical treatment.

Heart To examine the heart, the doctor first palpates, or feels, the chest with his hand to detect any abnormal beats or thrills, buzzing vibrations that accompany

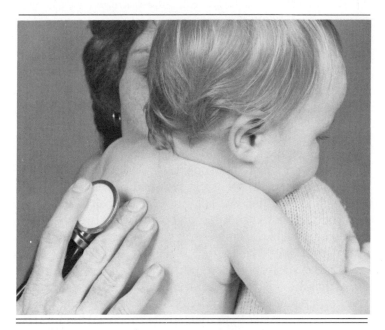

The doctor listens to both the heart and lungs with the stethoscope. Depending on the age of the child, he may need the parent's help.

heart murmurs. Then he listens with the stethoscope. Since the doctor can't hear anything if the child is crying, it's important that she be kept quiet and content for this part of the exam. Because the heart makes several kinds of sounds as it pumps blood through the body, the stethoscope is specially designed to pick up all of them.

The bell-shaped part of the instrument picks up low-pitched sounds and is held lightly against the chest for best results. The bell is especially useful for picking up the low-pitched sounds of innocent heart murmurs. Such heart murmurs are called innocent because they are not associated with heart disease and because children usually "outgrow" them without treatment.

The diaphragm, or flat-shaped part of the stethoscope, is for higher-pitched sounds and is pressed firmly against the child's chest. With this part of the stethoscope the doctor listens for heart rate—the number of beats per minute—and heart rhythm—whether steady or irregular. Then he moves the diaphragm to five different positions on the chest, which are roughly equivalent to the outline of the heart beneath, called the cardiac silhouette. Heart sounds are very complex, and they are tricky to listen to. There are two major heart sounds, each with two components. And each sound has a location where it's heard best.

Lungs In order to examine the lungs fully, the doctor first observes the chest and then listens to both the chest and back with the stethoscope. By looking at the chest, the doctor can check to see if it is symmetrical, as it should be as the child breathes. Actually, though, the bellies of infants and young children move in and out as they breathe more than their chests do. Nonetheless, the chest should remain symmetrical with breathing.

The doctor counts the number of breaths, or respirations, that the child takes per minute. Normal respiration in a young child is about 20 to 30 breaths per minute. (Newborns breathe faster than that, adults much slower.) As the child breathes, the doctor looks at his nostrils for any abnormal signs of flaring or widening that would indicate a breathing difficulty. He also listens for abnormal breathing sounds, such as grunting or wheezing. Other clues to lung and breathing problems are found in the fingers. Fingers that have a clubbed shape (like the end of a drumstick) or are purplish in color (cyanotic) signal either a heart or breathing problem.

With the stethoscope, the doctor listens to the baby's breath sounds as she breathes in and out. He listens in several places over the front and back of the chest for the normal sounds of inspiration (breathing in) and any abnormal sounds that indicate infection, airway obstruction, or fluid in the lungs.

Percussion is sometimes used to complete the examination of the lungs. With this technique, the doctor uses the middle finger of one hand as a sounding board by tapping on it with the tip of the middle finger of the other hand. As he taps over the lung fields on the child's chest and back, he can interpret the sounds. Normally the chest should sound resonant, or a bit hollow. If large amounts of fluid accumulate in the lung or chest cavity, the sound becomes dull. If the lung collapses, the sound may become drumlike.

Eyes　Examination of the eyes includes general observation as well as examination with instruments. One of the first things the doctor does is to look the child straight in the eye. There is much to see. The doctor notes the size and shape of the rims of the eye sockets (orbits) and whether they are equal in size. He also examines the lids, noting their position; their movement; and whether there is any swelling, redness, or crusting that would indicate an infection or other problem. He may even examine the eyelids for troublesome eyelashes that grow crookedly toward the eye instead of away from it. Such lashes cause irritation of the eye.

The tear ducts and glands are checked for redness and swelling in the glands and overflow of tears from the ducts. Tear ducts are the tiny pinpoint openings at the innermost corners of the lower eyelids. Glands are located in the upper eyelids. From a position above the child's head, the examiner can look down to see if both eyeballs

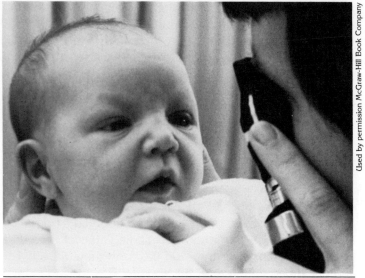

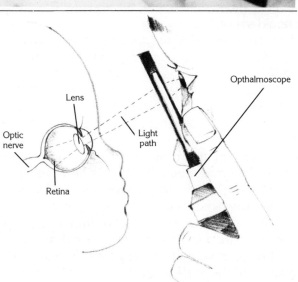

Optic nerve

Lens

Retina

Light path

Opthalmoscope

The doctor uses an ophthalmoscope to look inside the baby's eye. This instrument combines a light and a series of magnifying lenses, which allow him to focus on the structures inside the eye.

(globes) stick out the same distance from their sockets as they should.

Next comes examination with instruments. A penlight is used to test the responses of the pupils to light. Normal pupils shrink in size, becoming visibly smaller, when light is shined on them. Both pupils should reduce to similar size. If they don't, it might mean there has been damage to one of the nerve pathways leading to the eye.

To see inside the eye, the doctor uses an instrument called an ophthalmoscope, which consists of a light and a series of magnifying lenses that allow him to focus on various points on the inside of the eyeball. By dialing to different lenses and by varying the distance the ophthalmoscope is held from the child's eyes, the doctor is able to observe different parts of the inside of the eye. The red reflex, for example, is checked from a distance of about 6 to 12 inches from the eye, while the lens and retina are examined up close.

The red reflex is checked first. If you have ever driven on a dark country road at night and surprised an animal with your headlights, you probably saw its eyes shine red in the darkness. When the doctor shines the light into the baby's eyes looking for the red reflex, that is just what he sees. The pupils appear to be red because the light from the ophthalmoscope bounces off red blood cells flowing through the transparent inner lining of the eye (retina). When the doctor sees red, it means there are no major obstructions present, such as cataracts or tumors.

Moving close to the eye, the doctor then examines the lens located in the front of the eyeball. It is the job of the clear, or crystalline, lens to focus images. Both lenses must be checked to be sure they are unobstructed and in place.

Using the ophthalmoscope to look inside the eye is something like looking inside a shiny Christmas ornament. The retina, or inside lining of the eye, is shiny, too. It is a delicate membrane made up of special nerve cells, called rods and cones, that make vision possible. Rods are for night vision. Cones are for color and daylight vision.

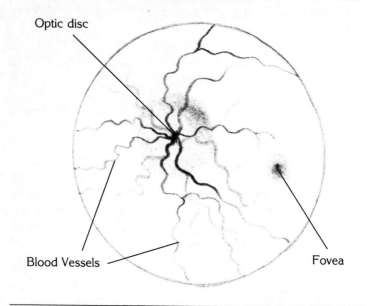

Optic disc

Blood Vessels

Fovea

The structures seen with the ophthalmoscope include the optic disc or optic nerve head (the entry of the optic nerve from the brain), the blood vessels that supply the retina, the retina itself, and the fovea, a small depression in the center of the retina, which is responsible for close vision.

Examining the retina, the doctor can see the optic nerve where it enters the back of the eye from the brain. This is called the optic disc or optic nerve head. He can also see a spot on the retina called the fovea. This is a little red depression in the center of the retina that is responsible for close vision. The doctor can see, too, the blood vessels that serve the retina and check them for any abnormalities such as clogging or narrowing. Such abnormalities are uncommon in infants and children, however. The most common abnormalities in children are malformations and tumors of the retina.

Vision is checked by having the baby follow an object with his eyes. In the early weeks, a baby's ability to track objects is limited, but by 3 months he can follow through a half circle—from a point near one of his shoulders all the way to the other one. This doesn't really tell the doctor how well the child sees, however. It says nothing about clarity of vision, distance vision, or color blindness. These important aspects of vision can't be checked accurately until a child is about 3 years old and can take an eye test based on his communicating what he sees.

Nose The examiner first looks at the shape of the nose and whether both sides are open. He may close one side at a time to see if the child can breathe through both sides. Children often put foreign bodies into their noses, which obstruct the passages and can also cause infection.

To look inside the nose, the doctor gently pushes the tip of the nose up and uses the otoscope (the same instrument used for the ear) to light the nasal passages. He can see the nasal septum, the thin membrane in the middle that divides the nose into two passages. He can also see the turbinates, the folds of tissue that act as filters to catch dirt and to purify the air we breathe. The nasal passage is lined with a special, moist mucous membrane that makes it efficient in picking foreign material out of the air that is breathed. The doctor checks to see if the nasal membranes are moist but not weeping and if they are the right color, rosy pink. A child with an upper respiratory infection or an allergy will have an increase in watery secretions and pale, swollen membranes that obstruct the nasal passage. If a bacterial infection occurs, the secretions become thick and yellow or greenish in color. A child with severe allergic runny nose may develop polyps, benign growths, in the nasal passage.

Mouth and Throat (Pharynx) Using a disposable wooden tongue depressor, the doctor checks the inside of the child's mouth carefully for sores, bumps, and color. (Most children enjoy this part of the exam about as much as they enjoy having their ears poked at, which is to say not at all.) The gums, tongue, and the inside of the mouth (buccal mucosa) should be pinkish and uniform in color.

If there are teeth, the doctor checks them, too. Teeth

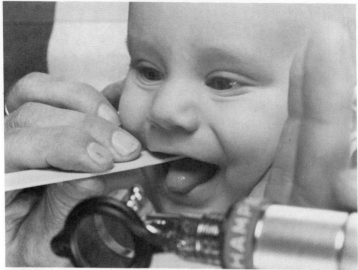

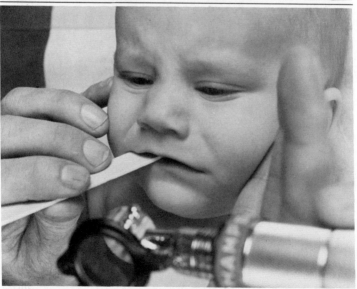

The mouth is examined using a wooden tongue depressor and a bright light. In addition to getting a good look at the gums, tongue, tonsils, and mucous membranes, the doctor tests the gag reflex to be sure the child can swallow normally.

should be neither crowded nor too far apart. If they are, spacing of the permanent teeth will almost certainly be a problem. The teeth are also examined for incomplete development of enamel, a condition that can be caused by heredity, infection during pregnancy, or prematurity. Inflammation of the gums near the base of the teeth usually indicates poor dental care, as do gums that bleed too easily.

Using a penlight and a tongue depressor, the doctor checks the back of the mouth and throat. At the back center of the roof of the mouth (palate) is the uvula, a small tag of flesh. The tonsils, located on either side of the back of the throat, are checked for size and appearance. The tonsils can grow to be quite large during childhood, then become smaller with puberty. When they are infected, they become swollen and red.

With the tongue depressor, the examiner presses on the back of the tongue, a maneuver that tests the gag reflex and also permits a quick glimpse down the throat of an uncooperative child. In this way the doctor is able to determine that the child can swallow properly. The gagging is only for a split second and does the child no harm at all.

Ears   Looking into an ear is a lot like peering down the drain in your kitchen sink. It's dark down there and dark inside the ear as well. There's a bend in the ear canal much like the bend in the sink drain. And, as with the drain, there may be some debris in the ear. Sometimes before examining a child's ear the doctor has to clear away ear wax (cerumen) with a special loop or flush it out with a syringe of warm water or hydrogen peroxide.

Examination of the ear is the part that babies and children seem to hate the most, so they fuss and wiggle a lot. Toddlers especially fear it will hurt. Ironically, examination of a healthy ear is completely painless as long as the child holds perfectly still, so all the fussing and wiggling work against a smooth examination. Sometimes the doctor needs help from the parent to hold the child still. And sometimes he has to skip the ears entirely in a very uncooperative child. Although a healthy ear doesn't hurt when it is examined, an infected one may.

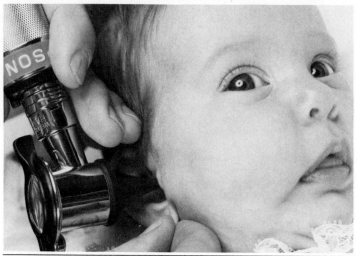

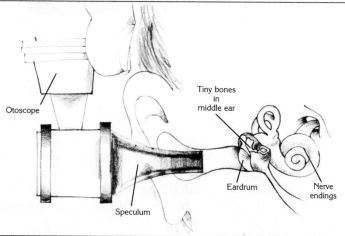

The ear is examined with an otoscope, an instrument that combines a light and a magnifying lens, which allow the doctor to see the eardrum. Pulling gently downward on the ear, he inserts the speculum partway into the ear canal. The anatomy of a normal ear is shown in the diagram. The eardrum, a thin membrane that stretches across the ear canal, is attached to three tiny bones in the middle ear. These tiny bones (ossicles) transmit the sound waves to the inner-ear nerve endings, the part that looks like a snail.

In order to see into the ear canal, the doctor uses an instrument called an otoscope. It consists of a light, a magnifying lens, and a cone-shaped viewer called a speculum. The viewers come in several sizes, and the doctor chooses the biggest one that will fit into the child's ear. A snug fit makes for greater comfort. In order to straighten out the canal for a clearer view, the doctor pulls the baby's earlobe down. With older children, the outer ear is grasped just above the lobe and pulled up and back to straighten out the canal. This is because the angle of the ear canal changes as the child's skull grows.

After straightening the canal, the doctor braces his other hand, the one that holds the otoscope, against the child's cheek or forehead. It is this steadying of the instrument that helps to make the process painless. As the drawing shows, the viewer/speculum goes only partway into the ear canal. There is no danger to the eardrum.

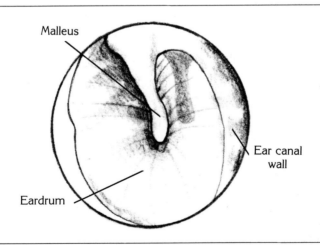

Malleus

Ear canal wall

Eardrum

The healthy eardrum (tympanic membrane) is a shiny, semitransparent membrane that stretches across the ear canal. The center is attached to one of the bony ossicles (the malleus), which transmits sound waves across the middle ear to the auditory nerve.

The doctor can see down the canal to the eardrum, or tympanic membrane. A healthy eardrum is shiny, semi-transparent, somewhat cone-shaped, and pearly gray in color. The examiner can see through a healthy drum to the middle ear beyond. A drum that has turned opaque is a sign of infection. So is a bulging drum or a drum that is perforated. Fluid behind the drum (serous otitis) indicates blocked Eustachian tubes, and when the fluid becomes infected it is called otitis media, middle-ear infection. Middle-ear infections are common in babies from age 6 months to 2 years and then again when they are older. Redness or change of color of the landmarks inside the ear also indicate infection. There are several landmarks inside the ear, and it takes years of training and practice to be able to identify them and interpret their appearance properly. Some doctors use an otoscope that has a plastic tube attached to it. By blowing gently through the tube as he examines the ear, the doctor can determine movement of the eardrum.

Looking inside the ear does not reveal how well the child hears. Hearing is determined by observing the child's reaction to sound and by following his speech development beginning at about age one year.

☆

Although the physical examination described in this chapter should be considered typical of well baby care, it shouldn't necessarily be considered a blueprint for your doctor's routine. Many doctors have developed special techniques of their own to carry out some portions of the examination. Also, the order of the examination will probably not be the same as listed here and every item will not always be included.

5
THE 2–4 WEEKS
CHECKUP

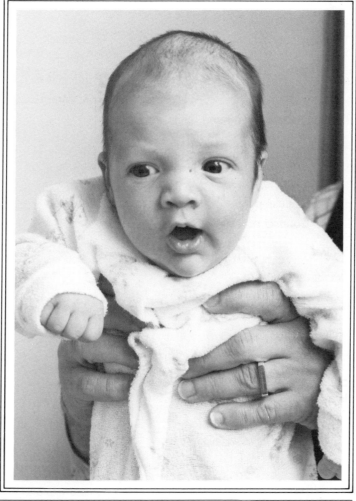

✓ CHECKLIST

2–4 WEEKS CHECKUP

Date _____

Procedures:

_____ Weigh and measure

Weight _____

Percentile _____

Height _____

Percentile _____

Head circumference _____

_____ Discuss weight and height gains on growth charts with parents

_____ PKU test if not done previously or if done before baby was 72 hours old; tests baby's ability to metabolize certain proteins

_____ Discuss parents' questions and concerns

_____ Counsel on safety

PHYSICAL EXAMINATION*

Special attention to:

_____ Urinary stream (boys)

_____ Vision

_____ Hearing

_____ Milestones in development (head control, ability to track object)

*The complete physical examination is described and illustrated in Chapter 4.

From 2 to 4 weeks of age is a good time for your baby's first checkup. It gives the doctor an early chance to see how things are going at home for you and the baby. The first procedure in the checkup is usually weighing and measuring the baby, done most often by a nurse or physician's assistant. This is one of the most important parts of the baby's health-care program. By regularly weighing and measuring the baby, you and the doctor can see exactly how he is growing and thriving. Weight gain should be steady at a rate of about 20 grams (nearly an ounce) a day for the first five months, equal roughly to 1½ pounds a month.

Your baby can also be expected to grow about an inch a month, 10 to 12 inches in the first year. The circumference of the head will grow about 5 inches in the first year, too, which shows his brain is growing rapidly, as it should be. Brain size increases dramatically in this first year of life; that's why it's important to measure the head periodically to check on the progress of brain growth.

A baby's head is his biggest part, bigger in circumference at birth than his chest. Measured from the top of his skull to the bottom of his chin, his head is equal to about 25 percent of his total body length. These proportions will change as he gets older. His chest circumference will catch up with his head when he's a year old, and his head will become proportionately smaller compared to the rest of his body as he grows older, too.

The baby's head is measured with a cloth or paper

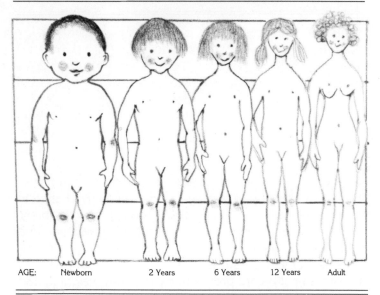

AGE: Newborn   2 Years   6 Years   12 Years   Adult

Head-to-body proportions change markedly from birth through adulthood. At birth a baby's head represents fully one fourth of total body length. The head becomes proportionately smaller as the child grows older. The adult head is only one eighth of total height.

tape. How it's done is important. The tape has to go around the biggest parts—the bump at the back of the head and the bony ridges over the eyebrows. The nurse may measure more than once to be sure the final figure is exact. Body length is measured by gently stretching the usually diaper-less baby out on the examining table. Sometimes the table has a built-in measuring device; otherwise the baby's length is marked with pencil on the paper that covers the table, then measured and recorded.

Next comes the weighing. Perfectly contented babies often become insulted and agitated at this point in the checkup. It may have something to do with the unstable surface of the scales. The slightest movement from the baby sets it in motion and probably makes him feel insecure. It is unlike any other surface he normally comes in contact with. In any case, most babies settle down again when they're removed from the scales. Weighing is most often done with the diaper on. When an extremely accurate weight is required, as with a premature baby, the weight of the diaper is taken into consideration.

Weight is measured and recorded in grams, height and head circumference are recorded in centimeters, and

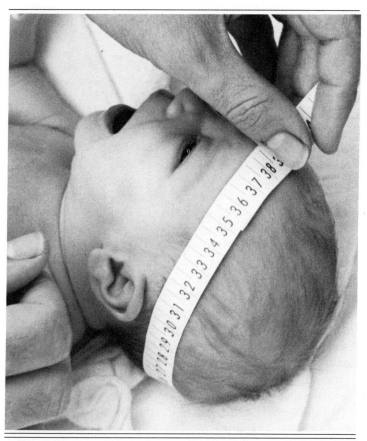

With a cloth or paper tape the baby's head is measured around its biggest parts—the bump at the back and the bony ridges over the eyebrows.

all three become an important part of your baby's permanent records. The nurse or physician's assistant will be glad to convert the figures to more familiar pounds and inches for you and will probably even record them that way on the slip of paper or booklet you may be given to take home with you. Later, the doctor will discuss the baby's gain in weight and length and plot out his progress for you on a standardized growth chart.

$$1 \text{ kg} = 2.2 \text{ lbs}$$
$$31 \text{ gm} = 1 \text{ oz}$$
$$2.5 \text{ cm} = 1 \text{ in}$$

There are several growth charts for weight, length/height, and head circumference available to doctors. Charts are classified according to age and sex—girls from birth to 36 months, for example. Charts are published by a number of sources, like the National Center for Health Statistics, and are constantly being revised. Most were developed by weighing and measuring large numbers of children regularly over a short period of time. Charts are provided at the back of this book so that you can plot your own baby's growth after each well baby checkup.

Although the weighing and measuring provide a good opportunity for you and the doctor to see how well your baby is doing physically, beware of the "numbers game." The numbers recorded for your baby's height and weight gain are important, but they don't tell the whole story. Babies grow and thrive according to their own built-in timetables. Small parents tend to have small children; larger parents, larger ones. If you look at the growth charts included in this chapter, you'll see that there is a *very wide range* of normal heights and weights.

Usually, but not always, height and weight fall into the same percentile. If a baby is in the sixtieth percentile for height and weight, it means that 40 percent of children are taller and heavier than he, whereas 60 percent are smaller and weigh less. Babies are little people, not little machines, so, although gains in height and weight are usually steady, they are not always precise. Some months he'll gain more weight than length. And vice versa. Illness can cause a temporary interruption in growth, but the baby usually catches up with an extra growth spurt to make up for the lapse.

Measurements of body length, weight, and head circumference are taken at each checkup and plotted on growth charts like the ones shown on the next four pages. The charts provide a visual comparison of the child's rate of growth to the normal range, shown in percentiles. For each measurement—head circumference, weight, and length— the 50th percentile, or average rate of growth, is represented by an extra heavy black line. Figures A and B show sample records for a 15-month-old boy (shown as dotted line). This child stayed close to the average (50th percentile) for length but was slightly underweight (25th percentile) for the first 12 months. This imbalance between length and weight is further highlighted by plotting length versus weight (Figure B, bottom). Between 6 and 12 months of age the boy's length-to-weight ratio fell as low as the 10th percentile for male children. His head circumference (Figure B, top) was always close to average. Figures C and D show sample records for a 15-month-old girl. Her rate of growth—length, weight, and head circumference—were all above average (75th to 90th percentile range). Her length-to-weight ratio (Figure D bottom) shows an almost perfect balance between her rate of growth and her weight gain. (Charts courtesy of Ross Laboratories, Columbus, Ohio.)

BOYS: BIRTH TO 36 MONTHS
PHYSICAL GROWTH
NCHS PERCENTILES*

NAME _____ RECORD # _____

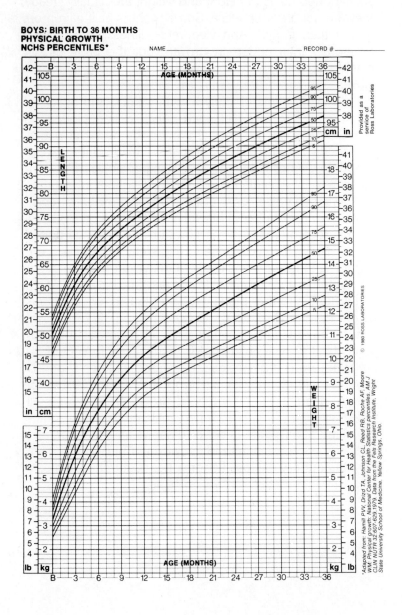

*Adapted from: Hamill PVV, Drizd TA, Johnson CL, Reed RB, Roche AF, Moore WM: Physical growth: National Center for Health Statistics percentiles. AM J CLIN NUTR 32:607-629, 1979. Data from the Fels Research Institute, Wright State University School of Medicine, Yellow Springs, Ohio.

A

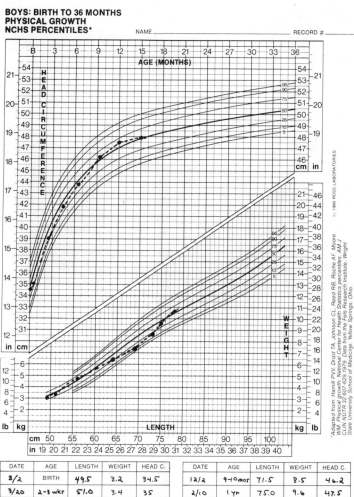

BOYS: BIRTH TO 36 MONTHS
PHYSICAL GROWTH
NCHS PERCENTILES*

NAME _____ RECORD # _____

DATE	AGE	LENGTH	WEIGHT	HEAD C.
3/2	BIRTH	49.5	3.2	34.5
3/20	2-3 wks	51.0	3.4	35
4/28	2 mos	58.0	4.8	39
7/8	4-5 mos	64.0	6.4	41.8
9/9	6-7 mos	69.0	7.3	43.7

DATE	AGE	LENGTH	WEIGHT	HEAD C.
12/2	9-10 mos	71.5	8.5	46.2
2/10	1 yr	75.0	9.6	47.5
5/5	15 mos	78.0	10.6	48

Preferable to cow milk during the first year
SIMILAC® WITH IRON   ADVANCE®
Infant Formula   Nutritional Beverage

For milk-sensitivity
ISOMIL®
Soy Isolate Formula

ROSS LABORATORIES
COLUMBUS, OHIO 43216
DIVISION OF ABBOTT LABORATORIES USA

G105 January 1980

*Adapted from: Hamill PVV, Drizd TA, Johnson CL, Reed RB, Roche AF, Moore WM. Physical growth: National Center for Health Statistics percentiles. AM J CLIN NUTR 32:607-629 1979. Data from the Fels Research Institute, Wright State University School of Medicine, Yellow Springs, Ohio.

© 1980 ROSS LABORATORIES

B

GIRLS: BIRTH TO 36 MONTHS
PHYSICAL GROWTH
NCHS PERCENTILES*

NAME_____ RECORD #_____

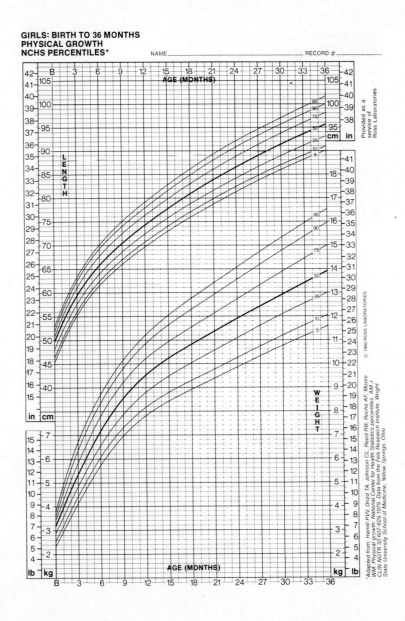

C

GIRLS: BIRTH TO 36 MONTHS
PHYSICAL GROWTH
NCHS PERCENTILES*

NAME _____ RECORD # _____

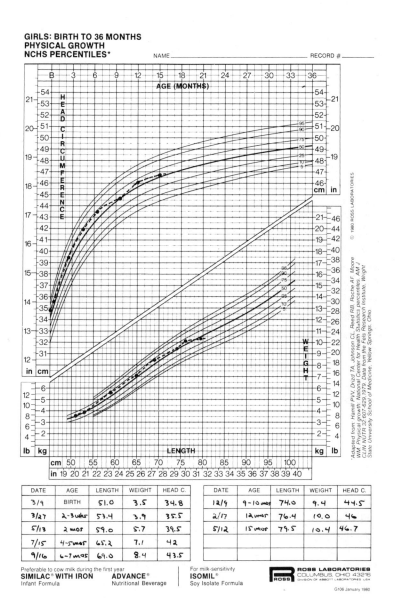

© 1980 ROSS LABORATORIES

*Adapted from: Hamill PVV, Drizd TA, Johnson CL, Reed RB, Roche AF, Moore WM. Physical growth: National Center for Health Statistics percentiles. AM J CLIN NUTR 32:607-629 1979. Data from the Fels Research Institute. Yellow Springs, Ohio. State University School of Medicine. Wright

DATE	AGE	LENGTH	WEIGHT	HEAD C.
3/9	BIRTH	51.0	3.5	34.8
3/27	2-3 wks	53.4	3.9	35.5
5/13	2 mos	59.0	5.7	39.5
7/15	4-5 mos	65.2	7.1	42
9/16	6-7 mos	69.0	8.4	43.5

DATE	AGE	LENGTH	WEIGHT	HEAD C.
12/9	9-10 mos	74.0	9.4	44.5
2/17	12 mos	76.4	10.0	46
5/12	15 mos	79.5	10.4	46.7

Preferable to cow milk during the first year
SIMILAC® WITH IRON   **ADVANCE®**
Infant Formula   Nutritional Beverage

For milk-sensitivity
ISOMIL®
Soy Isolate Formula

ROSS LABORATORIES
COLUMBUS, OHIO 43216
DIVISION OF ABBOTT LABORATORIES USA

G106 January 1980

D

THE PHYSICAL EXAMINATION

When the doctor arrives, she may be carrying a clip-board with your baby's medical record on it, which will show how he was doing at the time of his discharge from the hospital, how much he weighed then, whether he is breast- or bottle-fed, and whether or not there were any problems with the delivery. Her first question will probably be "How are things?" or "Are there any problems?" This is because she wants to know if there are problems that need to be discussed right away. Answer honestly. If some of the problems are yours, not the baby's, tell her about them. There will also be time later, after the physical examination, to talk about your problems and concerns.

If you say everything's going pretty well, the doctor will proceed with the examination, which always begins the same way, even though different doctors have different techniques and a different sequence. She'll begin by just looking at the unclothed baby. With boys, a diaper is usually draped loosely over the genital area as a defense against his natural urination reflex. The doctor is observing his skin, his color, how he moves and behaves. On his back, the baby frequently keeps his head turned to one side. The arm and leg on that side then automatically stretch out, giving him the appearance of being in a fencing position. Called the tonic neck reflex (TNR), this is normal. It disappears at about age 4 months and should not be present by 6 or 9 months.

The doctor will probably ask whether or not you think the baby can see and hear. Vision is checked by placing an object in the baby's line of vision (about 8 inches from his face) and then moving it to the midline, or center of the body. Sometimes the baby is too sleepy or too fussy to pay attention, but normally he will follow the object with his eyes, and sometimes his head, to his midline but no farther. This shows he can see an object at the expected distance and follow it briefly, which is just right for his age. Normal babies can also discriminate color at the age of 2 weeks. It

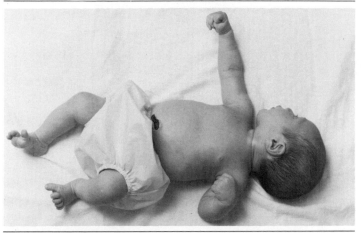

On his back, the baby frequently keeps his head turned to one side. The arm and leg on that side normally stretch out, giving him the appearance of being in a fencing position. This is called the tonic neck reflex (TNR).

is normal for babies of this age not to be able to focus their eyes all the time and to appear to be crosseyed occasionally.

The doctor checks hearing by making a clapping sound, snapping her fingers, or ringing a bell near the baby. There are several responses a baby makes that indicate he has heard the sound. He may startle. Or he may stop all activity and become suddenly still, as if listening intently, or his eyes may widen in surprise. This proves only that the baby hears somewhat loud noises, though, for the sounds made by the examiner are all much louder than the softest sounds a normal infant is expected to hear. This is not, then, a full test of hearing. Another flaw in the hearing test is that normal babies get used to noises and stop responding to them. So if the doctor has to snap her fingers or ring the bell more than once, the baby may not respond—not because he can't hear but because he has habituated to the sound.

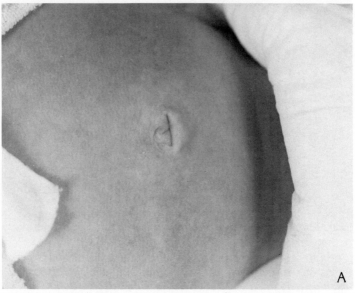

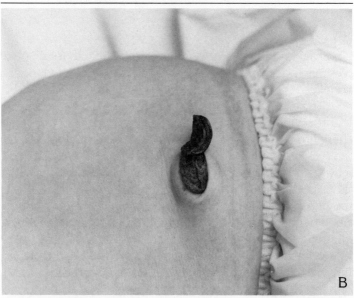

At age 3 weeks a baby's umbilical cord stump may (A) or may not (B) have fallen off. While the average is about 10 days to 2 weeks, 3 weeks or more is not unusual.

Next the doctor will perform a thorough physical examination, much like the one described in Chapter 4. She
will start with procedures that are least disturbing to the
baby and that require the least amount of handling (examining hands, necks, and underarms) and work up to the
others (abducting the hips; looking into the ears, nose, and
mouth with lighted instruments). She will listen to his heart
and lungs; feel his abdomen; examine his head, spine, neck
and genitals. Circumcision, if it was performed, should be
just about healed by now, and the umbilical cord stump
may have fallen off. If your baby is a boy, you should try to
observe his urinary stream whenever possible during these
first few weeks of life to be sure that it is strong and steady,
as it should be, with no dribbling or straining, which might
indicate a urinary-tract infection.

The doctor will want to check milestones in development that the baby should normally have reached by now.
She wants to be sure he is doing things reasonably on time.
Some of these things she can test for herself—head control, for example. For others, like smiling and cooing, she
may have to ask for your observations. Remember, though,
that there is a wide range of normal times concerning when
babies do various things. They have their own timetables on
these matters, just as they do with growing. You can,
however, help your baby's development by providing stimulation. Talking to him constantly, for example, helps him
to learn to socialize and vocalize. Providing him with visual
stimulation, such as mobiles and the right toys at the right
times, helps him to keep on schedule developmentally.

MILESTONES IN DEVELOPMENT ± *

Motor/Physical
- Holds head up briefly
- Follows object with eyes

Social/Personal
- Smiles

*The plus-or-minus sign indicates that your baby may reach developmental
milestones earlier or later than what is indicated here as "average." There is a wide
range of normal growth in child development.

Language/Communication
• Makes throaty noises

Motor/Physical   You can see changes in your baby almost daily. His neck muscles are getting stronger. Placed on his tummy, he moves his head to one side or the other to avoid smothering. This is a normal reflex and one that is reassuring for parents to know about. He can also lift his head briefly, as if to take stock of his surroundings. As mentioned previously, he can see an object held in his line of vision and follow it with his eyes for a short distance.

Social/Personal   He may already be smiling real smiles—as opposed to grimacing from gas pains—but he's still not much of a socialite, mostly because he sleeps much of the time.

Language/Communication   Although he communicates most of his needs by crying, he has also begun to make other throaty sounds occasionally. He listens to the sound of your voice and seems able to distinguish it from other voices. He regards your face when you put it close to his. It is good for you to relate to him this way, *en face* ("face-to-face," from the French), but be sure that when you do, you protect your eyes by holding both your baby's hands gently in your own. You can suffer serious eye injuries from your baby's uncontrolled arm movements. He still keeps his hands in a closed-fist position most of the time, however, so there is less danger from his fingernails now than there will be later.

NUTRITION

Breast milk or formula are all a baby needs for the next few months. Generally, doctors don't approve of changing a baby's formula unless he seems truly not to be thriving on it or is allergic to it. Both circumstances are rare. Commercial formulas are for the most part very similar to one another and there is nothing to be gained by switching them, although sometimes parents feel a change will solve unrelated problems like fussiness. It won't.

Water is an important part of your baby's diet, too. On

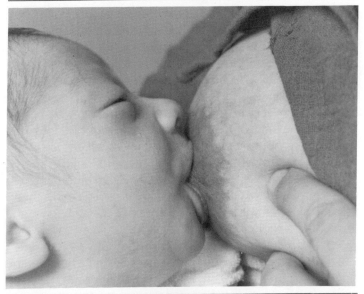

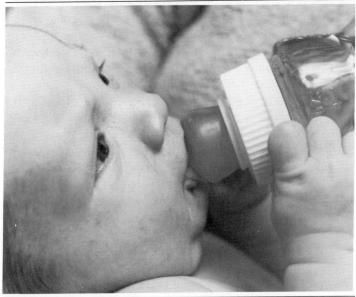

*Breast milk or formula are all a baby needs for the
next few months. Semisolid foods are not usually introduced
into the diet until age 4 months at the earliest.*

warm days when you feel thirsty, you can bet your baby does as well. He should be given small amounts of plain water from time to time.

Solid foods are not usually introduced into the baby's diet at this time because he isn't physically ready to handle them. His mouth and tongue are expert only at sucking. That works well with milk, but it's a disaster with solids. They get pushed out of his mouth and dribble down his chin. You're not feeding him so much as scooping up the spills. His gastrointestinal tract isn't ready for solids either. It is unable to digest proteins others than those contained in milk. Some parents suggest introducing solids early, thinking mistakenly it will help their baby sleep through the night. It will not. Sleeping through the night is related to age and weight, not to the kinds of foods in the baby's diet.

Iron, Vitamins, and Fluoride   At this checkup the doctor may prescribe iron, vitamins, and flouride to supplement your baby's diet. She may prescribe one, two, or all three at once. Then again, she may not prescribe any of them yet because there is some flexibility—and even some controversy—about the timing. A lot will depend, too, on whether your baby is breast- or bottle-fed and whether he was premature or had a low birthweight.

Everybody needs iron, especially children. They grow very fast during the first year, and their cells—especially their red blood cells—need iron to grow. Without enough iron, babies may develop iron deficiency anemia, and when it's severe enough, there isn't enough iron to make red blood cells. Even slight deficiencies of iron can cause problems. It has been suggested that mild deficiencies may be implicated in behavior and school achievement problems in older children, for example.

While everybody agrees that children need iron, nobody agrees about when supplements should begin. Although it is believed that all healthy full-term babies are born with enough iron stores to last until they are 4 or 5 months old, some doctors think iron supplements should begin at birth; others, at 2 months; and still others, at 4 months. Since 1970, the Nutrition Committee of the American Academy of Pediatrics (AAP) has recommended iron supplementation from one or more sources for *all* children to begin no later than 4 months of age, 2 months if the baby was premature. Since breast milk contains small but very well-utilized amounts of iron, supplementation is not usually prescribed for breast-fed babies until they are 4 to 6 months old. Meanwhile, some babies are fed iron-fortified formula from birth.

Sources of iron are iron-fortified formula, iron-fortified cereal, and iron drops. The doctor will prescribe what she thinks is best for your baby. If iron drops are prescribed, keep no more than a month's supply on hand. Iron can be fatal to young children when accidentally taken in large amounts. It is also important that the daily dose never be more than the doctor prescribes.

Vitamins may become part of your baby's diet now, too, usually A, C, and D. Vitamins are natural, organic substances found in plants and animals. They're essential in small amounts to the body's healthy functioning. The emphasis here is on *small amounts*. Great megadoses of vitamins don't produce healthier bodies and babies. In fact, they are very dangerous. An overdose of vitamin A, for example, produces acute illness in babies, along with abnormalities of the brain, bones, and skin.

Introducing vitamins to your baby's diet is the doctor's job and not something you should try to do on your own. Never give your baby more vitamins or bigger doses than are prescribed. Unfortunately, there are cases reported in the medical literature of parents who have unintentionally made their children very sick and even retarded their growth by giving them too many vitamins. Vitamins A and D especially must be supervised by a doctor. Vitamin D is usually prescribed for breast-fed babies at this first office visit because breast milk contains very little of this vitamin, which is so important to healthy bone formation. When you give your baby drops of vitamins, fluoride, or iron, place the dropper well inside his mouth at the back of one cheek before you squeeze the drops out. Otherwise, his sucking reflex will cause the liquid to dribble back out.

Fluoride is a nutrient found in very small doses in many foods and in slightly larger amounts in seafoods. It creates tougher, more decay-resistant tooth enamel, and hence, fewer cavities (called "dental caries" by the medical and dental professions). The correlation between fluoride in drinking water and the prevention of tooth decay was confirmed by United States Public Health studies of community water supplies conducted between 1935 and 1950. Fluoride has reduced dental caries by as much as 60 percent in communities where there is fluoride in the drinking water.

Like Goldilocks' porridge, the daily dose of fluoride must be just right. Too little results in less than the desired protection. Too much can mottle, pit, and discolor the enamel on the child's teeth. So, like vitamins, fluoride supplements must be supervised by a doctor, who will take into consideration the American Academy of Pediatrics' recommended dosage schedule along with the amount of fluoride, if any, in your community's water supply. If your baby is breast-fed, he may be fed very little water, and the full recommended daily dose of fluoride might be prescribed. One last thing—although the AAP strongly recommends fluoride in precise amounts for all babies shortly after birth, it also recognizes that fluoride can be started as late as 6 months of age and still provide satisfactory results.

That brings us back to the beginning. Sometime, maybe today, your doctor will prescribe iron, vitamins, and fluoride for your baby.

PARENT CONCERNS

(These are only some of the concerns parents have at this time. Be sure you have yours written down to discuss with the doctor. *Remember there's no such thing as a dumb question.*)

Blocked Tear Duct A single tear duct is located on the inside of each eye near the bridge of the nose. It is the job of this tiny tube to channel internally a slow, steady drip of tears from glands located at the top of the eye. This internal drip is continual in everybody. (When you cry, too many tears are produced to be processed by the ducts, so the tears spill over.)

A baby's tear ducts are smaller than the point of a pin, so no wonder they become clogged. When they do, the affected eye tears constantly. Sometimes there is a pussy discharge, in which case a prescription ointment or drops may be necessary. Often, though, the blocked duct clears up by itself. There is also a massage that your doctor can show you. It involves placing your forefinger carefully at the corner of the baby's eye near the bridge of the nose, then applying pressure while moving your finger down about a half inch.

Bowel Movements   Babies may have as many as seven or eight bowel movements (stools) a day, with the average between two and eight. Breast-fed babies don't usually have as many as bottle babies, and the consistency of the stool is usually softer. Many babies have a bowel movement just after a feeding, caused by a reflex in the gastrointestinal system. Some babies take up to 15 minutes to have a BM, producing a little bit at a time, but it all counts as one movement.

Some parents are concerned because their babies seem to strain and fuss and become red in the face when they are moving their bowels. Consider for a minute how tough it would be for you to have a BM without your feet touching the floor. Now imagine that, worse still, you're sitting propped up with several folds of diaper under your bottom. You can see why a certain amount of straining and fussing is normal.

Diarrhea is defined as frequent runny or watery bowel movements and should be reported to the doctor. The danger with diarrhea is that the baby will become dehydrated, something that can happen quickly with a small baby.

Constipation has nothing to do with how often your baby moves his bowels, but rather what those bowel movements look like—hard and like pellets. Constipation, too, should be reported to the doctor, as should any bowel movements that are bloody or contain mucus.

Chin Trembling   You've probably noticed that when your baby's feelings are really hurt and he's having a good cry, his chin trembles between sobs. This is normal, but the cause is unknown. A certain amount of tremulousness is common in newborns.

Colic   Sometimes babies up to 3 months of age have long, unexplained crying periods when they also pass a lot of gas with their legs drawn up as if they were in pain. Although the exact cause is uncertain, excessive air swallowing, anxious parents, and a tense household seem to play a role. So first of all, try to be as relaxed as possible with your baby during mealtimes. Burp him frequently. If you use bottles, be sure the nipples aren't too large or too small. Feed him in a semisitting position and keep him that way for about a half hour after each feeding. Most of all, try to keep calm. He'll outgrow it, and you'll survive it. Colic rarely persists after 3 months of age.

Consoling   After you're sure she's dry, fed, and burped, try consoling your fussy baby in stages rather than picking her up right away. Remember that she has consoling mechanisms of her own and that if you rush to pick her up every time she whimpers, you will quickly train her—or she you—to expect it. Dr. T. Berry Brazelton of Harvard University suggests you begin by putting your face close to hers, then talking to her. If that doesn't calm her, place your hand on the baby's stomach. Next fold her arms together over her tummy and hold her hands in yours. The next step is swaddling her in blankets. Still no success? Now pick her up. Simultaneous walking, rocking, and talking are the last resort. Remember, too, that it's normal and okay for babies to cry. All babies cry in the first six weeks.

Cradle Cap   The medical term for cradle cap is seborrheic dermatitis, a scaling and crusting of the scalp that commonly appears in the first month of life. Although the cause is unknown, poor hygiene may contribute to the severity of the condition. There may be involvement elsewhere on the body, too, that is hard to distinguish from the usual diaper rash. If the condition develops and persists despite the fact that you are shampooing the baby's hair regularly one, two, or three times a week and rinsing well, the doctor may suggest either an antidandruff shampoo or a special prescription ointment to be applied directly to the affected areas. Don't use either special shampoos or ointments unless they have been prescribed by the doctor, though. Brushing the scalp with a soft-bristled brush may help. Rubbing oil into the scalp will make it worse.

Crib Death   The medical term for crib death is Sudden Infant Death Syndrome (SIDS). It is an as-yet unexplained killer of babies in the first year of life, as many as 10,000 of them each year in the United States. There is no way either to predict or to prevent these deaths, 90 percent of which occur between ages one and six months. Although the cause is not known and the cure has not been found, it *is* certain that parents are in no way responsible.

Home monitors are now available for infants who have been identified as at risk for SIDS, but monitors should not be purchased by parents except under the direction and supervision of a doctor or medical center. Although most manufacturers of monitors do not sell their products directly to parents, a few do.

Fussy Periods   It's normal for babies to cry. It's one of the things they do best, after all, and it's also their only means of communication in the first few weeks of life. Some newborns cry as much as two and a half hours a day. Your baby may have regular crying jags that even come at the same time of day. Once you've made certain that he is warm, dry, and not hungry, you can let him cry some. It won't hurt him as long as he isn't left for really long periods. His crying will lessen as he gets older.

Rashes   Although they all look pretty much alike to the untrained eye, rashes actually come in a variety of types, are caused by a number of factors, and can happen in the best of families. Most babies get rashes in the diaper area from time to time. They are usually caused by the baby's being kept too long in wet or soiled diapers. Plastic pants make the condition worse because they seal in the moisture.

A urine-soaked diaper is a great place for bacteria from the skin and the diaper to break down urea (the principal ingredient in urine) into ammonia. Ammonia is very irritating to the skin. Similarly, soiled diapers contain bacteria that break down and irritate the skin, especially if the bowel movement was abnormal, as with diarrhea.

Any rash that doesn't respond to careful washing, frequent diaper changing, and a protective coating of zinc oxide or an ointment such as A & D should be evaluated by a doctor. Ointments should be applied lightly to the skin and massaged in well so they can't be felt.

Besides bacteria, other possible causes of diaper rash include yeast (fungus) infection, allergy, or seborrheic dermatitis—the same one that causes cradle cap. The common yeast infection goes by three fancy names—candidiasis, thrush, and moniliasis—and can affect the baby's mouth as well as his bottom. This is because many of us, including babies, carry the yeast around in our gastrointestinal tracts, where it looks for opportunities to cause trouble.

Diaper rashes can also be caused by allergy, although rarely. For proper treatment a laboratory culture may need to be done to determine the exact cause of the rash.

Siblings   If you have brought your baby home to one or more brothers and sisters, they may greet the new arrival with anything from anxiety to anger. Although this is a natural reaction on their part and one you should be sympathetic to, remember that it can be dangerous for the new baby to be left unattended with a jealous brother or sister who hasn't had time yet to sort out his or her feelings. Older children need a lot of love, attention, and understanding from you at this time. It will help to try not to change their routine too much. It's probably not a good time to introduce a new bed or move the child to another bedroom. It may also help to let the child "assist" you in caring for the baby. Siblings can help with the bath, smooth on ointment, get a clean diaper, and so on.

Sleep Patterns Your baby still sleeps most of the time, but there are subtle differences in his sleep patterns. He stays awake for slightly longer periods now. Whereas two and a half hours was about the longest he was awake at any one time as a newborn, he is sometimes awake now for a little over three hours at a time. He is steadily increasing the number of hours he can sleep without waking, too. He's nowhere near ready to sleep through the night regularly, but he's practicing, working toward six hours at a stretch, compared to just over four hours when he was brand new. Normally, he will match his sleep patterns to the rest of the family's in time.

Remember that some of his wakeful periods occur in the middle of the night and that if he shares your room, he may be encouraged to socialize then, disturbing your sleep.

Travel When is it okay for new babies to travel? Check with your doctor to be sure, but usually the baby is ready when you are. If you're planning a car trip, be sure you have a dynamically crash-tested car seat. Take along a first aid kit with a rectal thermometer, petroleum jelly, and zinc oxide or other ointment for diaper rash. If the purity of the water supply will be unreliable, take ready-to-use, pre-mixed formula or a container of sterile water, boiled several minutes, with a tight-fitting lid.

So long as you are there and his meals are regular, the baby will be a super traveler—camper, hiker, airplane, or car passenger. Remember that neither adults nor children should travel by plane when they have upper respiratory tract infections (head colds, ear problems), as these make you really uncomfortable in a pressurized cabin.

Your baby is not old enough yet to be carried in a back carrier because he can't support his own head. Any hiking will have to be done with a front, sling-type carrier. Wherever you take him, don't bundle him up too warmly. Dress him in as many clothes as make you comfortable on any given day. Try to imagine how you would feel on a warm spring day dressed in wool trousers and a down parka, for example. It's not uncommon, either, to see new parents tenderly holding babies who have blankets pulled down over their faces. If you've ever tried to breathe with a blanket over your face, you know it's not easy. Babies are just little people; their needs are the same as yours.

REMINDERS

Safety Topics   Baby equipment and furniture, car seats. See Chapter 3.

Alcohol, Cigarettes, and Drugs   Although alcohol consumed in moderation by a nursing mother has traditionally been thought to do no harm to the nursing infant, this may not really be the case. Unborn babies *are* harmed by their mothers' drinking. It has been shown that fetal growth and development are adversely affected when mothers are alcoholic and that the babies may be born with fetal alcohol syndrome (FAS). The syndrome includes facial abnormalities, low birthweight, faulty central nervous system (CNS) development, and mental deficiency. There is no agreement yet on how much, if any, alcohol is safe for a pregnant woman to consume before risking a defective child, but some researchers are convinced that even relatively small amounts can do damage.

After birth, babies continue to be at a critical period in their physical growth and mental development and may, therefore, be at risk for continued damage by alcohol. If a nursing mother drinks alcoholic beverages, detectable amounts of alcohol appear in the breast milk. What isn't known is the amount of alcohol that is dangerous for the baby. It is known, though, that alcohol adversely affects the mother's milk supply. Although small amounts of alcohol have been said to aid in the letting down of breast milk, animal and human studies have shown just the opposite. The milk supply is actually interferred with and possibly reduced when alcohol is consumed in amounts well within the range of social drinking.

Like alcohol, cigarettes may affect babies both before and after birth. Babies of smoking mothers weigh less and are smaller all over than those of nonsmoking mothers. More than forty scientific studies, reporting on over half a million babies born since 1957, show that the more a mother smokes, the greater will be the reduction in the baby's birthweight. Smoking also increases the risk of prematurity.

If you smoke, you are also a health hazard to your newborn. First, you pollute the air he breathes. Children of smoking parents are more likely to suffer from bronchitis and pneumonia in the first year of life. Second, and more serious, a positive association has been found between Sudden Infant Death Syndrome (SIDS) and smoking during pregnancy plus exposure to smoke (passive, involuntary smoking) after birth.

Finally, nursing babies get nicotine through breast milk, with a direct-dose relationship between the number of cigarettes smoked and the amount of nicotine in the breast milk. Although all the effects are not known, two cases of nicotine poisoning in babies 3 and 6 weeks old have been reported. Suspected but not proved are measurable deficiencies in physical growth and intellectual and emotional development in the children of smoking parents.

If you can't give up smoking, you can at least provide certain safeguards for your baby. Set aside a room for him, preferably his own, where no one is allowed to smoke. And never smoke when you handle him.

Drugs, as in medications, are transmitted to babies through breast milk, and some may be dangerous to him. If you are taking a prescription medication, check with your baby's doctor to see if you need to stop breast-feeding temporarily. Among the drugs that are known contraindications to nursing are chemotherapeutic agents, anticoagulants, narcotics, radioactive material, cathartics, antithyroid drugs, iodine, and bromides. "Recreational" drugs are also transmitted through breast milk and range from undesirable to dangerous for both parent and child.

Babysitters   The search for responsible babysitters can be frustrating. Family members or close friends who have babies of their own are a good choice, especially in the beginning, when most new parents are uneasy about leaving their babies in someone else's care. Reliable sitters can also be found through a professional agency. Although they are usually expensive, they often have undergone screening by the agency.

One dependable method is to advertise in your local newspaper for a sitter and then interview her in her own home, which will tell you a great deal about her. Once you've found a sitter, make the house rules clear, whatever they are. With teenagers, it might be no visitors while sitting, or one friend (the same sex) on approval, or no smoking.

Leave the name, address, and phone number where you will be. If you can't be reached, leave the number of a responsible friend (with the friend's permission). Leave all the necessary emergency numbers in a prominent place—doctor, police, poison information center. Give the sitter specific emergency instructions. For instance, in case of fire she should: (1) Get the baby. (2) Leave the house. (3) Phone the fire department from a neighbor's home. Finally, responsibility works both ways, so be home when you say you will. If there is an unavoidable delay, call the babysitter and let him or her know.

Immunizations Have you been fully immunized against polio? Your baby will get his first dose of oral vaccine (TOPV) at the next well baby checkup. There is a slight chance—one in five to ten million—that you could contract the disease at that time if you haven't been immunized. Even though that seems like a small risk, there are baby clinics that routinely caution parents about it.

Sun Your baby should not be exposed to the sun until he is at least 2 months old. A newborn's skin is very delicate and easily burned.

Toys Babies need something interesting to look at from their cribs. Hang colorful pictures on the walls of your child's room, and use printed crib sheets and colorful crib bumper pads to provide visual stimulation for him. Mobiles are ideal toys for this age, but they should be interesting from the baby's point of view. Some mobiles that look wonderful to the buyer are really a disaster to the little person who's flat on his back looking up. Get flat on *your* back if you have to and check it from your baby's perspective before you buy it.

Some brands of "jungle gyms" designed for cribs have been recalled by the manufacturer because babies have strangled in them. If you have any doubt about the safety of toys or equipment you plan to buy, call 1-800-638-8326/8333 toll free for further information from the U.S. Product Safety Commission. Be sure you have the name of the manufacturer and the model number when you telephone.

HOW ARE THINGS?

Sometimes it takes the patience of Job to be the father of a newborn. Two things in particular may be hard for you to deal with. First, the baby takes up a lot of time you and your wife used to have together. You're both tired and getting less sleep than usual, too, which doesn't help. Second, if you want to share equally in the parenting, it may not be easy. Your time with the baby is necessarily limited to the number of hours you're at home, fewer than your wife, in the beginning, at least.

If the baby is breast-fed, you may begin to feel you don't contribute anything important to the baby's needs. By nursing, your wife is not only developing a strong maternal bond with the baby, but she is also providing him with his only source of nourishment. You may feel left out, inadequate, even jealous. And then you may feel guilty for having those feelings. But they aren't shameful; they're quite normal, and most new fathers have them. Recognizing them is an important step in being able to deal with them. It's important to tell your wife how you feel, too. Just talking about it will help a great deal.

Also, don't minimize the importance of the things you can do for the baby. You can change him, hold and comfort him, and talk to him. All of these are crucial to his development and wellbeing. Later, when he begins to eat solid foods, you can feed him. Much later, when he goes off to college, you get to pay the tuition.

NEXT CHECKUP

Your baby's next checkup will be in about a month, when he is 2 or 3 months old. Don't wait that long to get in touch with the doctor if the baby is having a problem or seems not to be thriving. Here are some of the milestones in development you should be looking for in the meantime. (See the next chapter for details.)

- Lifts head higher (on tummy)
- Follows with eyes, maintains eye contact
- Responds to voice
- More alert
- Vocalizes
- Smiles responsively

RESOURCES

Ross Laboratories provides a number of booklets written for parents and available to them exclusively from pediatricians' offices. Some titles include *Becoming a Parent, Caring for Your Baby, Breast-feeding Your Baby,* and *The Phenomena of Early Development.*

Your pediatrician's office or well baby clinic will have a number of other helpful free publications as well.

Tel-Med Tel-Med, Inc. is a national nonprofit organization that provides free tape-recorded health information by telephone, in some cases on a 24-hour basis. Each licensed Tel-Med program—300 of them in 40 states—has a library of more than 300 tapes (also available in Spanish), many of which concern care of the newborn as well as infant and child health care. From three to five minutes in length, each tape is screened for content by doctors and other health professionals, and the tapes are updated yearly.

Tel-Med is sponsored by different organizations in different communities—the county medical organization, local hospital, Blue Cross/Blue Shield, state university, and United Way, for example. In some cases the phone listing may be under the name of the sponsoring organization rather than Tel-Med itself. If you are unable to find Tel-Med, call your local county medical organization for help. Tel-Med national headquarters are at 22700 Cooley Drive, Colton, California 92324, telephone 714-825-6034.

In order to make use of Tel-Med tapes, you need to send for the free catalog of titles. Each tape has a number for use in requesting tapes from Tel-Med operators.

Sullivan, S. Adams, **The Father's Almanac.** Garden City, N.Y.: Doubleday & Co., Inc, 1980.

6
THE 2–3 MONTHS CHECKUP

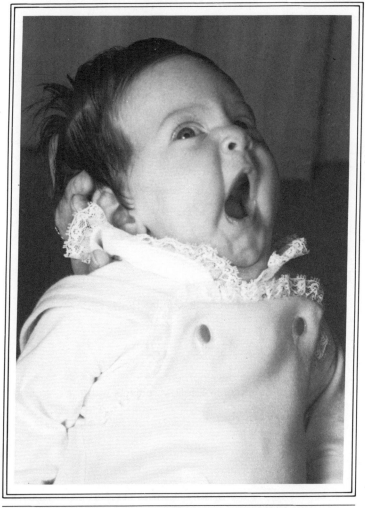

✓ CHECKLIST

2–3 MONTHS CHECKUP

Date _____

Procedures:

_____ Weigh and measure

Weight _____
Percentile _____
Height _____
Percentile _____
Head circumference _____

_____ Discuss weight and height gains on
growth charts with parents

_____ Immunizations _____ DTP (diphtheria/tetanus/
pertussis) #1
_____ TOPV (trivalent oral
poliovirus
vaccine) #1

_____ Discuss nutrition

_____ Ask about parent concerns

_____ Counsel on safety

PHYSICAL EXAMINATION*
Special attention to:

_____ Hearing

_____ Vision

_____ Milestones in development
(better head control, follows objects with eyes, smiles)

*The complete physical examination is described and illustrated in Chapter 4.

Many doctors and clinics choose age 2 months for the second well baby checkup for a very practical reason. Immunizations are recommended at that age. (See the immunization schedule that follows.) So, since the child has to come to the office to get them, it's a convenient time to examine her and see how things are going. It isn't necessary, of course, to give the shots at exactly age 2 months. In fact, it may not be possible to administer them then if the baby is ill at that time or the parents are unable to schedule the visit for some reason. In any case, your baby will probably have this checkup sometime between ages 2 and 3 months, if not exactly at 2 months. Some pediatricians even schedule office visits at both 2 *and* 3 months of age, and a few immunize children a week or two earlier than that.

THE PHYSICAL EXAMINATION

The doctor or nurse practitioner will probably perform a physical examination much like the one described in Chapter 4. Special attention will be paid to head control (head lag) as the baby is pulled by her arms to a sitting position from a lying-down position. There is a dramatic difference in head control between 2- and 3-month-old babies. The 2-month-old shows little head control, although the head doesn't flop back quite so much as when she was a newborn. She is able to lift it slightly as she is pulled to sit. Once in a sitting position, she should be able to hold her head up quite well, although it bobs forward frequently. A 3-month-old, on the other hand, shows only slight head lag when pulled to sit. He also has good head control when sitting, although his head bobs forward occasionally.

The 3-month-old has also reached a milestone in length, having increased his length at birth by about 20 percent. That means if he was 20 inches long when he was born, he's now almost 24 inches long.

At the end of the examination your baby will get her first "shots," immunization against diphtheria, tetanus (lockjaw), pertussis (whooping cough), and polio. The American Academy of Pediatrics' *Red Book: Report of the Committee on Infectious Diseases,* updated regularly, recommends that *all* children be immunized against these and other diseases beginning at this age.

Reaction to the shots, if any, is usually mild—a low-grade fever within 12 to 24 hours, some fussiness, and poor feeding. Most serious reactions, including high fever, occur within 24 hours.

CALLING THE DOCTOR

Call the doctor immediately if the baby has any of the following *abnormal* reactions:

- Fever of over 101–102°F, taken rectally
- Convulsions (involuntary twitching, rigidity)
- Excessive listlessness or drowsiness (baby unable to be wakened)
- More than 24 hours of fussiness and unconsolable crying
- Pronounced redness, hardness, or swelling at the site of the injection (may indicate infection or localized allergy to shot)

Fever, or "running a temperature," is the body's response to either a viral illness or a bacterial infection. Because this first immunization involves the introduction of weakened viruses *and* bacteria into the baby's body, it is only natural to expect the body to respond with fever. A fever of up to about 101° isn't usually a cause for concern.

Higher than that, though, is too high for babies less than 3 months of age for anything but a short period of time.

For most parents the first rectal temperature is the scariest, but it needn't be. Shake the thermometer down to below 97°F. Do this over a soft surface like a carpet or a piece of stuffed furniture. That way the thermometer won't break if it slips out of your hands. Coat the bulb of the thermometer with petroleum jelly from a sterile tube. Place your baby face down on your lap or other surface. Spread his buttocks and *gently* insert the thermometer to a distance of 1 to 1½ inches, no more. Hold his buttocks together with one hand and keep him as still as possible until the temperature has had a chance to register, in about three to four minutes. A normal rectal temperature is usually around 99.6°F, about a degree higher than by mouth.

IMMUNIZATION

The body's immune system consists of a special set of cells called lymphocytes. They are able to recognize invading bacteria, viruses, and other harmful cells and then manufacture antibodies to fight and destroy them. Although lymphocytes can be found circulating just about everywhere in the body, there are four major "command posts" for their manufacture and distribution. These are the bone marrow, the lymph nodes, the spleen, and the thymus gland. The thymus is extremely important to the baby's immunity process. Later, when the child is about 5 years old, it shrinks.

Normal babies are born with fully developed but unchallenged immune systems. They have all the mechanisms necessary to make their own antibodies against disease, but they have had no occasion yet to use them. For the first few weeks of life babies have natural immunity to some diseases, immunity that they received from their mothers through the placenta (transplacentally). But this immunity first diminishes and then disappears fairly quickly. Breast-fed babies have immunity to intestinal dis-

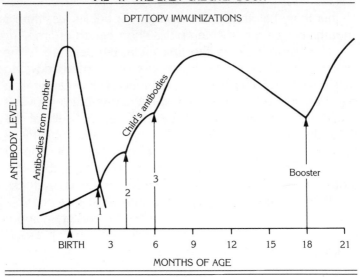

DPT/TOPV IMMUNIZATIONS

*Antibodies against disease that cross the placenta
from mother to baby decline rapidly in the first
two months of life. A series of three immunizations is
begun at age 2 months and is timed to give maximum
protection in the first year. A booster is given at
age 18 months to maintain the antibody level.*

orders from their mothers' milk. There is some evidence that they are also protected from severe diarrhea.

In Grandma's day, the only way to build up immunity to childhood diseases such as measles, mumps, and whooping cough was to actually catch the disease. If you survived, you were immune from catching that disease again for the rest of your life. Unfortunately, though, all of these highly communicable diseases can produce serious complications and even death in some children. This is true of the first set of diseases your baby will be immunized against. Each disease is devastating to a small baby.

Diphtheria Diphtheria is a highly infectious disease of the nose and/or throat caused by a kind of bacteria spread by secretions from the nose and throat of carriers and victims of the disease. Children under the age of 15 years are the most susceptible, and since 10 percent of diphtheria victims die, you can see how important it is for your baby to be vaccinated against this disease. In its early stages diphtheria may resemble a common cold or sore throat. But left untreated, it causes tissue destruction of affected areas along with production of dangerous toxins (poisons) that can be spread throughout the body by the bloodstream, causing damage to and dysfunction of the heart, nervous system, and kidneys.

RECOMMENDED IMMUNIZATION SCHEDULE FOR NORMAL CHILDREN

2 months	DTP (diphtheria/ tetanus/ pertussis)	TOPV (trivalent oral poliovirus vaccine)
4 months	DTP	TOPV
6 months	DTP	TOPV*
1 year	No immunizations (formerly smallpox vaccination)	
15 months	MMR (measles/ mumps/rubella)	
18 months	DTP	TOPV
4–6 years	DTP	TOPV
14–16 years	Td** (repeat every 10 years)	TOPV

*Optional

**Combined tetanus and reduced-strength diphtheria
Adapted from *Report of the Committee on Infectious Diseases.*
American Academy of Pediatrics. 18th ed. Evanston: 1977.

Tetanus (Lockjaw) Tetanus, or lockjaw, is caused by bacteria that grow in contaminated wounds and produce a toxin that affects the central nervous system (CNS). Principal sources of contamination of wounds are soil and dust, animal or human waste, and unsterile stitches in a wound. When a wound becomes infected by tetanus it can cause pain, muscle spasms, and rigidity around the area of the wound, which may last for weeks but eventually get better. This is called *localized tetanus.* Untreated, it can lead to *generalized tetanus,* the most common form of the disease. Symptoms are stiff neck, difficulty swallowing, and headache in the early stages, followed by uncontrolled and painful muscle spasms that affect internal organs as well as body extremities and the face. The name lockjaw, in fact, comes from the disease's effect on the face, which loses mobility and appears frozen into a grimace.

Pertussis (Whooping Cough) Like diphtheria, whooping cough is a highly contagious bacterial disease. It can be serious—especially when it affects children under the age of 5 years. Although immunization has significantly reduced the incidence of this disease, it has not completely eradicated it. In some patients immunization is apparently impermanent and incomplete because cases have been reported in vaccinated people. The disease begins with a mild cough that becomes increasingly severe and is often, though not always, characterized by a distinctive whooping sound. The whoop is heard when the victim struggles to breathe in after an uncontrolled fit of coughing so severe that it can also cause the face to turn red or blue, bulging eyes, and vomiting.

Poliomyelitis (Polio) Polio is caused by any one of three types of virus, each of which causes a different form of polio and all of which are contagious. A mild case of polio may present almost no symptoms at all, while the disease in its most severe form can cause paralysis, permanent crippling, and death. There is no cure for polio once it has been contracted. The only way to control it is by continued use of the very effective oral polio vaccine. The vaccine contains three strains of virus to combat each of the three types of polio. Two doses are recommended for babies, at ages 2 and 4 months. A third dose at age 6 months is optional. Your doctor will recommend the third dose if you live in an area of high risk where there is a past history of polio outbreaks or if your baby is breast-fed. The vaccine may not be as effective in breast-fed babies, so a third dose is indicated.

The Vaccines Vaccines provide immunization against diseases by introducing the disease into the body in either a highly weakened or killed form to produce antibodies and immunity, but not sickness. In addition to DTP and polio, vaccines are available for measles, mumps, and rubella (German measles) and will be given to your baby when she is older. DTP is injected into the baby's upper thigh muscle. The injection site is important, and the thigh is chosen because it is the largest muscle a little baby has and is least likely to suffer damage to a major nerve because of the injection. Polio vaccine is given orally. A few fruit-flavored drops are placed in the baby's mouth. Although most babies smack their lips over the polio vaccine, they hate the needle in their thigh. All health professionals are sensitive to the fact that it is the first deliberate hurt a baby suffers. Some doctors like to give their own shots, while others prefer to have an assistant do it for them. It is always done at the end of the examination. One pediatrician remarked that the whole profession survives only because babies have such poor memories. "Otherwise," he philosophized, "they'd all be out gunning for us when they grew up."

There are two kinds of immunization. The previously mentioned vaccines—DTP and TOPV—provide *active immunization* for your baby. That means they cause her body to create antibodies against the various diseases so that she becomes immune to them for relatively long periods of time. For some diseases, though—hepatitis, for example— no vaccine has been successfully developed. Active immunization isn't possible, but by administering antibodies from an immune person (called immune serum globulin/ ISG) another person can receive *passive immunization.* Passive immunization is not as dependable as active immunization. It isn't always effective, and protection doesn't last very long. Its duration varies between one and six weeks.

Risks and Reactions   In the first two days after a DTP shot, many children develop a slight fever and crankiness. Some develop soreness and swelling in the thigh where the shot was given. More serious side effects are rare. Only about one out of every 7,000 immunized children develops a very high fever, a convulsion, or a crying spell that lasts for several hours. In about one out of every 100,000 doses encephalitis (inflammation of the brain) or brain damage may occur. As you can see, the shots are not entirely risk-free, but the benefits far outweigh the risks, because the diseases the shots are designed to prevent are deadly, especially in unprotected babies.

There are no side effects from oral polio vaccine, but there is a risk estimated to be one in every 5 (some say 10) million doses. A person who receives oral polio vaccine or who comes in contact with someone else who has received it recently may develop paralytic polio and may even die. Slight though the risk is, some well baby clinics advise the parents and relatives of babies who will be immunized to be sure that their own polio immunization is up to date.

Contraindications Routine immunizations should not be given to babies who are very sick or who are running a high temperature. The doctor may also decide to delay the shots if the baby is now in good health but had some medical problem in the first few weeks of life. Convulsions after the first DTP shot indicate that the child should not receive a second pertussis shot. She should be given DT (diphtheria/tetanus) only for the rest of the series. Prolonged, unconsolable crying or screaming after a DTP shot indicates that the next pertussis shot should either be withheld or be given in a half dose for the rest of the series.

Immunizations are available either free of charge or at reduced cost from your local health department. Before arranging to have them done there, though, check with your baby's doctor. Some doctors are uncomfortable about accepting followup responsibility for shots they did not administer themselves. If your baby had an adverse reaction, for example, it might well occur after the health department's regular business hours and would become your doctor's responsibility. Other doctors don't mind this at all and even suggest the health department to their patients with tight budgets.

Don't forget to enter this DTP/TOPV immunization in the permanent record form provided at the back of this book. Although your baby's doctor keeps records, it is extremely important that you have records of your own. That way, if you move, change doctors, or need quick access to your records, you'll have them. You would be surprised at how many times during the course of a year you need to know what shots your child has had. You won't be surprised to hear how your doctor's office responds when you ask them repeatedly to supply that information.

At the end of the examination, after your baby has been immunized, the doctor or nurse will probably tell you to telephone if she shows any of the abnormal reactions listed at the beginning of this chapter. You will also be instructed about what to do for fever. Doctors usually tell parents to telephone the office or clinic if the fever reaches 101° or 102°F taken rectally. You'll no doubt be advised to buy either "baby" aspirin or Tylenol, and you will be given instructions for their use. Be sure to write those instructions down if the doctor doesn't. Both aspirin and Tylenol will help bring down a fever, but neither should be used unless the doctor prescribes them.

The generic name for aspirin is acetylsalicylic acid. It is available in tablets of reduced strength for children, often flavored artificially to mask its naturally bitter taste. A tablet or part of a tablet, whichever is prescribed, must be crushed between two spoons and diluted with water before being given to a baby. Acetaminophen is the generic name for Tylenol. Like aspirin, it reduces fever. Your doctor may leave it up to you to choose between the two, or he may have a definite preference. Tylenol is available in liquid form, which makes it easier to administer to a small baby. Aspirin is not. It's very important to give either medication in exactly the right strength and dose and spaced the right number of hours apart. Be sure to follow the doctor's instructions and read the instructions on the label as well. Keep all medications in a safe place.

The 1970 Poison Prevention Packaging Act requires that all prescription medications for adults and children be dispensed in containers with childproof caps. This includes aspirin and Tylenol, even though they are not prescription drugs, because overdoses of either drug can cause death in babies and young children. Despite this protective legislation, not all prescription drugs are dispensed in childproof containers. Pharmacists are allowed to sell drugs in non-childproof containers at the request of customers who first sign a release form stating that they specifically requested regular caps instead of child-resistant safety caps. It is not unusual for customers to make this request, so there is still a lot of medicine leaving United States pharmacies in containers that are potentially dangerous to babies and young children.

The doctor may also discuss sponge bathing as a method of reducing fever in your child, although some doctors don't think it is useful. This involves placing the undressed baby into a bath of lukewarm, tepid, *not cold* water and sponging him off. The bath water should be slightly warmer than room temperature, allowing blood vessels on the surface of the skin to dilate (widen) and give off heat. Cold water would create a cold shell (the skin) around a hot core and make things worse. The baby will object to the bath because fever makes the body play tricks on the mind. Although he is actually very warm, he feels cold and wants to be bundled up.

MILESTONES IN DEVELOPMENT ± *

Motor/Physical
- On tummy, lifts head
- Fists no longer tightly clenched
- Holds object in hand briefly
- Follows object with eyes

Personal/Social
- Maintains eye contact
- Smiles

Language/Communication
- Coos, laughs, and squeals

---

*The plus-or-minus sign indicates that your baby may reach developmental milestones earlier or later than what is indicated here as "average." There is a wide range of normal in child development.

What a difference a month can make! The differences in development, in fact, between a 2- and 3-month-old are so striking that both ages will be discussed in this section, illustrated by photographs of a 2-month-old girl and a 3-month-old boy. All the developmental milestones just listed are common to both ages but with quite a difference in level of performance.

Motor/Physical   Placed on her tummy, the 2-month-

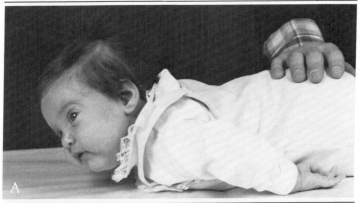

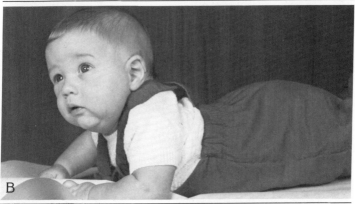

At age 2 months Anna (A) can lift her head to an angle of about 45 degrees, while 3-month-old Eric (B) can lift his head to an angle of almost 90 degrees. He can lift his chest off the examining table as well.

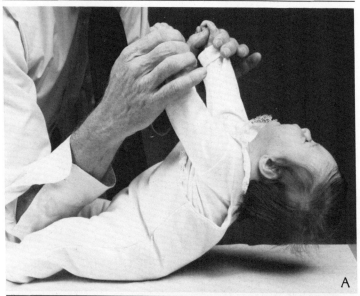

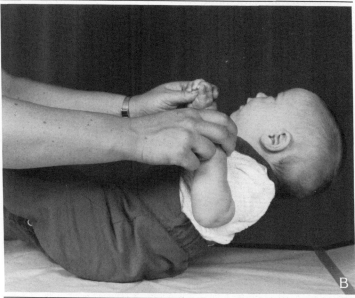

A 2-month-old's head lags behind her body when she is pulled to a sitting position (A). A 3-month-old shows improved head control as he is pulled to sit (B).

old can lift her head to an angle of about 45 degrees, but for only brief periods of time. The 3-month-old lifts his head for sustained periods and can lift his chest up off the examining table briefly as well. The 2-month-old's head still lags behind her body when she is lifted by her arms from a lying-down position, which means she continues to need head support when she's handled. The 3-month-old does not. His head control is dramatically improved. Supported in a sitting position, they both bob their heads up and down, the 2-month-old more than the 3-month-old.

The 2-month-old has begun to relax her hands at times from the tight-fistedness characteristic of newborns and younger babies. The 3-month-old, in contrast, keeps his hands in a relaxed, open position. Further, he has begun to bring them together and move them up over his chest and face, where he enjoys gazing at them intently, even though he's not quite sure where they came from. This is a characteristic pose of a 3- to 4-month-old and is considered to be a critical sign of normal development.

Both 2- and 3-month-olds have a distinct way of hold-

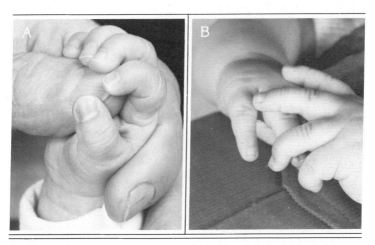

The 2-month-old (A) has begun to relax her hands from the tight-fistedness she showed at birth. The 3-month-old (B) keeps his hands in a relaxed, open position.

ing things. If you place an object in their hands, they hold it as if they were wearing a mitten, using the thumb as one unit and all four fingers together as the other unit in order to hold the object. This is called the palmar or "mitten" grasp. At neither age can a baby willingly let go of an object. He or she can only release it accidentally.

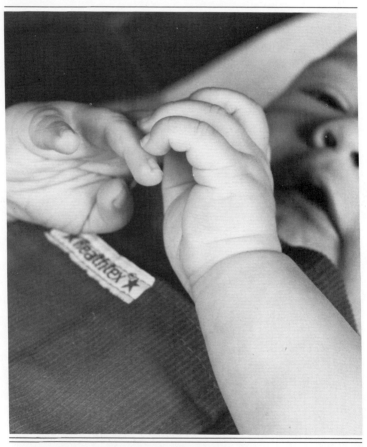

Hands together over the face is the typical pose of a 3- to 4-month-old and is a critical sign of normal development.

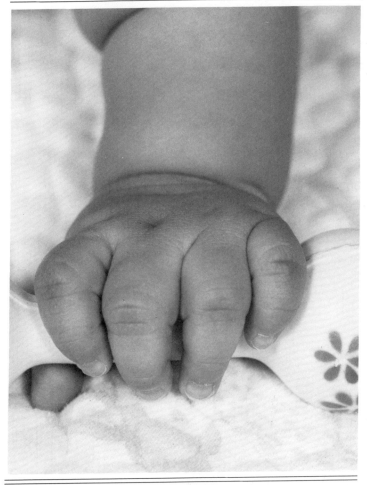

*The mitten grasp—all four fingers opposing
the thumb—is typical of both 2- and 3-month olds.*

The 2-month-old can't bear very much weight on her legs, whereas the 3-month-old loves to stand for brief periods, even though he is stiff at the knees, a characteristic of babies this age when they stand.

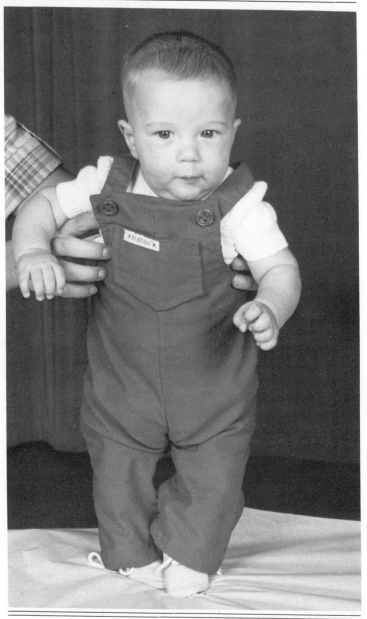

*At age 3 months babies love to stand for
brief periods and are typically stiff at the knees.*

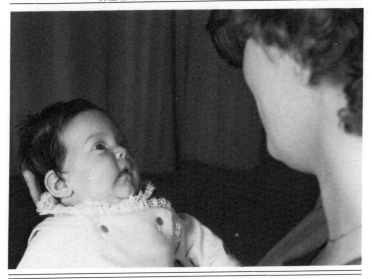

A 2-month-old attends (pays attention to) her mother. She will maintain eye contact for increasing periods of time as she gets older.

As for vision, if you place a brightly colored object above the nose of a 2-month-old and then move it down toward her shoulder, she'll follow it for a bit with her eyes before losing track of it. But she'll stop tracking it before it reaches her shoulder. Most 3-month-olds do better than that. They follow the object (ball or yarn pompom) from their nose to one shoulder and then through a semicircle all the way back to the other shoulder, although not necessarily with continuous, smooth motion.

A distinct difference between the two ages is the extent of their visual interest in small objects, such as a raisin. A 2-month-old pays no attention whatsoever to a raisin. It's as if it didn't exist. The 3-month-old notices it and pays attention to it for a little while before losing interest.

Personal/Social Smiling is a key development, one of the first clues that a baby is normal. By the age of 2 months, a baby should smile in response to attempts to get her to do so, such as smiling and talking to her, tickling her gently, and so on. A baby of that age who did not smile responsively would need to be evaluated further. By age 3 months, a baby not only smiles responsively, but he has also begun to use smiling as a social tool. You don't need to poke him to get him to smile. He smiles first in an effort to get your attention. About half of all 3-month-olds do that. A few 2-month-olds do it, too. Children of both ages can make eye contact with another person, but the 3-month-old maintains it for a longer period of time.

Socially, babies of both ages are real charmers. They recognize members of their own family. A 3-month-old has the wonderful knack of greeting a family member he hasn't seen in a while with a hundred-percent effort. He gets into it with his whole body—kicking of legs, waving of arms, big grin, and much panting and excitement.

Language/Communication   A 2-month-old is making continual progress in the area of communication. Although she still does more crying than anything else—it is, after all, her chief method of communication—she is beginning to make more kinds of noises, especially cooing, and she may even be laughing out loud. Her fussy periods are decreasing. The 3-month-old vocalizes even more and cries even less. He has learned to "talk" back when you talk to him, something you should do frequently, since it will be a great help in his speech and social development. Most 3-month-olds not only laugh out loud but actually squeal with delight.

NUTRITION

The nutrition message for this checkup is simple. No solids yet. No juice either. Although you may be tired of hearing it, it is nonetheless true that your baby at age 2 or 3 months still needs nothing more to thrive on than milk. The diet of a breast-fed infant is sometimes supplemented by now with vitamins C and D, iron, and fluoride. Formula, already fortified with vitamins, may be supplemented now with iron and fluoride. These supplements are discussed in the nutrition section of Chapter 5, "2–4 Weeks Checkup."

Before 1920, solids were seldom fed to infants before age one year. Over the next fifty years, recommendations were made that limited solids (cereals, strained vegetables, and fruits) be introduced at 6 months of age. Soon, solids were being introduced as early as age 6 weeks, and parents got into the spirit of the competition to see whose baby would get cereal first. It became a matter of misplaced pride and satisfaction for parents to be able to start their babies on solid foods at increasingly early ages. We now know, though, that a baby isn't physically ready for solids until about 4 months of age and that 3 months is absolutely the earliest that solids should be introduced. In the first place, before he is 4 months old, the baby doesn't know what to do with solids that are put in his mouth. His instincts tell him to suck, and when he does, the solids dribble back down his chin. Second, his gastrointestinal (GI) system isn't ready to process solid foods. He has no defense mechanisms yet in his GI tract to cope with the foreign proteins contained in foods other than milk. As a result, these proteins pass directly through the intestinal wall and into the body, where it becomes the job of the kidneys to pump them out. Unfortunately, the kidneys, too, are immature and not up to the task. This increases the chance of the baby's developing a food allergy. By waiting a little longer to add solids to his diet, these problems can all be avoided.

Like all disciplines, however, medical science is not immune from exceptions to its rules. And there are exceptions to the "no solids before 4 months" rule. Rice cereal, the least likely to cause allergy problems, is sometimes introduced quite early into the diet of a *very* hungry baby. By definition, a very hungry baby is one who is growing fast (documented by his growth chart), consistently drinks more than a quart of milk a day, and chews his fingers looking for more. Another exception is that some doctors suggest solids at 3 months, the earliest possible age they can be tolerated. Finally, a few doctors agree to solids even earlier than that, not because they approve of them but because they know they can't prevent it if the parents are really determined.

If you are one of those determined parents, you will want to be aware that there are some foods that should be avoided for the sake of your baby's health. Beets, carrots, and spinach should not be fed to babies less than 3 or 4 months of age. These vegetables are rich in nitrate, which can turn into nitrite in the bodies of little babies. The nitrite, in turn, affects red blood cells so that they can no longer carry oxygen throughout the body, causing a serious disease called methemaglobinemia.

Another food to avoid is honey, which should be withheld for the whole first year of life. This favorite natural sweetener has been implicated in cases of infant botulism poisoning. Botulism spores are not killed by the homogenizing process in the production of honey, and they may germinate into toxins in the baby's intestine.

PARENT CONCERNS

(These are only some of the concerns parents have at this checkup. Be sure you have yours written down to discuss with the doctor.)

Fussy Periods   At age 2 months, your baby's major method of communication is still crying. So it is normal for her to have regular, if fewer, fussy periods. She is telling you a number of things with her fussing—that she's sleepy, bored, hungry, wet, or wants some attention. By now you can probably tell which cry is which and respond accordingly. You may want to experiment by picking her up and socializing with her when she is not crying. That way you reinforce her good behavior rather than her fussiness.

Sleep Patterns   Most parents are interested in knowing when their babies will sleep through the night. Many do so on a regular basis at about age 4 months, and some begin to do so as early as 3 months. Meanwhile, your baby has probably progressed to only one feeding in the middle of the night because she has increased the number of hours she is able to sleep at one time. At 2 months, she sleeps for well over 6 hours at a stretch, and by 3 months, she will sleep more than 7 hours at a time. These long periods of sleep should occur at night, because by now the baby should have adopted the family's pattern of wakefulness during the day and sleeping at night.

Testicles (Testes)   It is normal for the testicles of infant boys to retract—or shrink back up toward the inguinal canal—from exposure to cold temperatures. This response continues throughout infancy and into childhood and adulthood. It is not normal, however, for one or both testicles to be up and out of the scrotum, or undescended, all the time. That condition should be evaluated by a physician.

REMINDERS

Safety Topics   Baby equipment. Safe handling. Unsafe toys. See Chapter 3.

Pets   Tell your doctor if you have a dog or cat at home. Both are commonly infected with a disease that can be passed along to humans. Mostly it affects older babies, but your doctor may want to check your baby for infection. See Chapter 13 for details.

Sunburn   A baby's skin is extremely delicate and sensitive to sun. It takes only a few minutes for skin to burn. Be sure he is well protected—cover over stroller or carriage, sun hat, covered arms and legs, umbrella over the infant seat—whatever it takes to protect him.

Travel   When you travel with your baby now, add aspirin or Tylenol to your medical kit, which should already contain a rectal thermometer, petroleum jelly, and ointment for diaper rash. Babies who have head colds or ear infections should not travel by airplane.

HOW ARE THINGS?

By the time your baby is 3 months old, he or she should fit nicely into your family. There should be a match by now between you and the child, meaning that even if your baby is somehow different from you and perhaps even different from what you expected, the baby is acceptable to you. Although this fitting or matching process is usually complete by age 3 months, that isn't always the case.

Some babies are vastly different from what their parents were expecting. Sometimes temperaments are a mismatch. The parents are warm and affectionate, but the baby seems distant and doesn't like to be held. Or the baby cries a lot and the parents are upset and even angered by the crying, although they try very hard not to be. Sometimes quiet parents are overwhelmed by extremely active babies. And, of course, the reverse is also true. Active, athletic parents may be puzzled by placid babies.

Mismatches *do* occur, and it's important to know that they do. It's also important to know that a mismatch is nobody's fault—not yours and certainly not the baby's. If your baby is 3 months old and you're still asking yourself where he came from and wishing you could turn him in for another model, you probably need some help, and your doctor can help you get it. Tell the doctor *now* if you are feeling mismatched. Many parents feel that way, and it's nothing to be ashamed or embarrassed about. Sometimes parents who don't get help find themselves physically hurting children they have been unable to accept, a situation that is as terrible for the parent as it is for the child.

NEXT CHECKUP
Baby's next checkup will be in two months, when he is 4 or 5 months old. Don't wait that long to get in touch with the doctor if the baby is having a problem or seems not to be thriving. Here are some milestones in development that you should be looking for in the meantime (see the next chapter for details). Baby

- Rolls over
- Has improved head control
- Holds object in hand for longer period
- Follows object with eyes better
- Recognizes familiar faces
- Turns toward sound
- Sleeps through the night

RESOURCES

Parents Anonymous (P.A.) is an international self-help organization founded in the United States and dedicated to child-abuse intervention. Help for parents in a crisis situation is available on a twenty-four-hour basis through the *P.A. hotline, telephone 1-800-421-0353.*Counseling is available through that number, as well as information about the caller's nearest P.A. group. There are groups in all fifty states and in a number of foreign countries as well. On weekends the hotline is answered by an answering service, but crisis calls are put through to a P.A. member.

7
THE 4–5 MONTHS CHECKUP

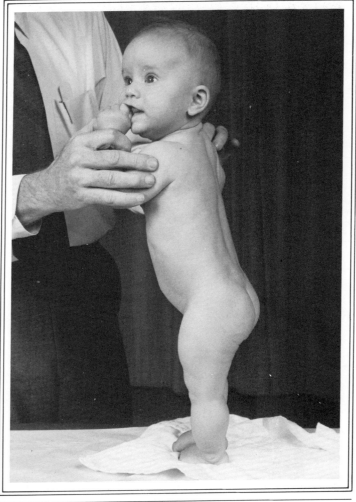

✓ CHECKLIST

4—5 MONTHS CHECKUP

Date _____

Procedures:

_____ Weigh and measure

Weight _____

Percentile _____

Height _____

Percentile _____

Head circumference _____

_____ Discuss weight and height gains on growth charts with parents

_____ Immunizations _____ DTP (diphtheria/tetanus/pertussis) #2

_____ TOPV (trivalent oral poliovirus vaccine) #2

_____ Discuss solid foods

_____ Discuss parent concerns

_____ Counsel on Safety

PHYSICAL EXAMINATION*

Special attention to:

_____ Vision

_____ Hearing

_____ Milestones in development (head control, ability to: roll over, grasp objects voluntarily, bear weight on legs, laugh out loud)

*The complete physical examination is described and illustrated in Chapter 4.

This checkup, like the previous one at age 2–3 months, was scheduled in part to accommodate your baby's immunization schedule. Unless he is off schedule for some reason, he will have his second set of immunizations at this checkup—DTP (combined diphtheria, tetanus, and pertussis) injected into his thigh and a second dose of TOPV (oral polio vaccine). When you return home, he will need to be observed for abnormal reactions to the shot, although it is unlikely he will have them now if he didn't before. Any of the following should be reported to the doctor's office immediately.

- Fever of over 101–102° taken rectally
- Convulsions
- Excessive listlessness or drowsiness
- Excessive fussiness for more than 24 hours
- Pronounced redness, hardness, or swelling near the injection site
- Breathing difficulties

After a DTP shot the development of a central nervous system (CNS) disorder, or thrombocytopenia (a blood disorder), or a prolonged spell of crying/screaming is usually attributed to the pertussis part of the DTP injection. If your child had these kinds of adverse reactions to his first immunization at the last checkup, pertussis will either be withheld entirely now or be reduced to half strength.

There are a number of interesting highlights associated with this checkup. The one you may have been waiting for is the introduction of solid foods into your baby's diet. In addition, this checkup comes at a point when your baby has turned a real corner in development. Most of his reflexes have disappeared, and he is accelerating his physical accomplishments. He is, or very soon will be, doing all of the following: rolling over, sleeping through the night, fussing less, holding his head up without help, and more. Even more exciting, his fine motor skills are beginning to develop, the ones that require his eyes and hands to work together. Evidence of this is his response to objects. Once satisfied with just looking at them, now he swipes at them in an effort to grab them. He has reached the "see it with the eye and grab it with the hand" stage. In addition to all these accomplishments, he's spectacularly good-natured. He isn't quite old enough yet to be wary of strangers, so he's probably very tolerant about being examined by the doctor, too.

THE PHYSICAL EXAMINATION

As usual, he'll be weighed and measured first. The average baby doubles his birthweight by 4 or 5 months of age, so your baby should weigh about twice as much at this

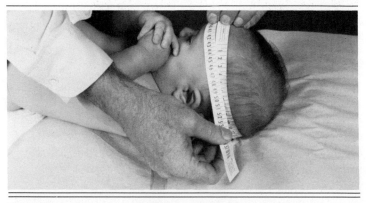

The first procedure in most examinations is weighing and measuring. Babies usually double their birthweight by 4 or 5 months of age.

checkup as he did when he was born. When the doctor arrives, he'll ask the usual "How are things?" and you, as usual, should be ready with your questions and concerns, preferably written down so you won't forget anything. Remember, there's no such thing as a dumb question.

The doctor may ask you questions, too, about the baby's eating, sleeping, and bowel movements, and about socialization within the family. If your baby still seems somehow not to fit in to the structure of your family, this would be a good time to mention it to the doctor. Most important, don't wait for the doctor to ask about something that concerns you, for she may not. Take the initiative and talk about what bothers you.

The physical exam will probably be a check of just about everything—skin and general appearance, head, eyes, ears, nose, throat, heart, lungs, belly, genitals, hips, neck, underarms, hands and feet, legs and arms, anus—the works. The complete physical examination is described and illustrated in Chapter 4.

In checking your baby's vision, the doctor should find

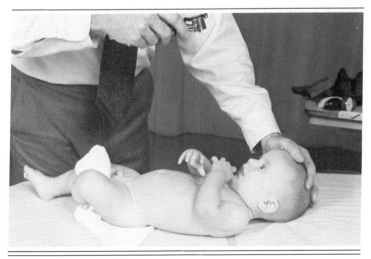

The 4-month-old can follow a light through a semicircle with his eyes.

that the baby can follow an object or a light 180 degrees, in other words, through a full semicircle. This can be done either with the baby in your arms or lying on his back. The doctor catches the baby's attention with an object and then moves it immediately to the side, to a point just over one of the baby's shoulders. He then moves the object in an arc all the way over to the baby's other shoulder. The baby should follow it with his head and eyes from one shoulder to the other in a smooth, continuous motion. You may remember that he could do that when he was 3 months old, too, but the motion wasn't necessarily smooth or continuous. Now it is. Also, 4-month-olds have full color vision.

The hearing check, only a rough estimate at best, is aided at this age by an additional clue. At age 4 or 5 months, babies should turn their heads or their eyes toward the sounds they hear. Younger babies startle, become still, or widen their eyes, but they don't turn their heads to try to locate the source of the sound. The 4- to 5-month-old does, even to a whispered sound. This is a test you can and should perform frequently at home. Moderate hearing losses can come and go with ear infections and should be evaluated by an audiologist.

During the course of the examination, the doctor will check the baby's motor activities to be sure he is accomplishing developmental tasks such as holding objects in his hands, lifting his head and chest up off the examining table when placed on his stomach, and keeping his head in line with his body when he's pulled to a sitting position.

MILESTONES IN DEVELOPMENT ± *

Motor/Physical
- Good head control
- On tummy, raises head and chest from examining table

*The plus-or-minus sign indicates that your baby may reach developmental milestones earlier or later than what is indicated here as "average." There is a wide range of normal in child development.

- Holds rattle in either hand
- Bears weight on legs
- Rolls over one way (usually tummy to back)

Personal/Social
- Smiles first to get attention

Language/Communication
- Laughs out loud, squeals, vocalizes

Motor/Physical　This is a big month for your baby developmentally. His nervous system has matured to the point at which voluntary behavior is replacing purely reflexive behavior. In practical terms, this means that when you place an object in his hand, he holds it because he wants to. Previously, his grasp reflex forced him to hold it, like it or not. Notice, too, how he holds his body. It's relaxed, no longer curled into a little ball with arms and legs folded close to his body. His hands have opened permanently from the closed-fist position. Both are signs of central and peripheral nervous system maturity. He is reaching out now with his body as well as with his mind.

All normal children follow a pattern of motor development that is a push against gravity. That is, first they sit, then crawl, then stand, and finally walk. In order to do any of this, of course, they must first gain control of their heads. At 4 months, a baby's head control is good. Pulled up by his arms when lying on his back, he keeps his head in line with his body as he reaches a sitting position. Head lag is either gone entirely or exists only slightly at the beginning of the maneuver. His head is steady as he sits. Head control is good enough so that he can be carried now in a back carrier instead of a front sling. And, having attained almost perfect head control, your baby is progressing to the next item on the development agenda—his body and extremities.

On his back, the baby assumes a pose typical of 4-month-olds (and some 3-month-olds). He brings his hands together over his face and holds them there, looking at them for long moments. He may even get a bald spot on the back of his head because of his fondness for this

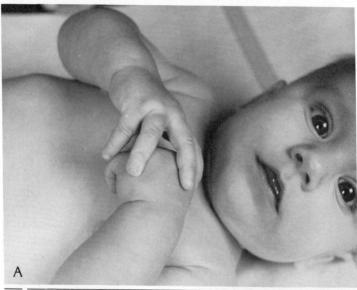

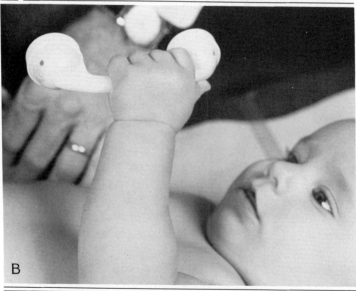

Typically, the 4-month-old brings his hands together over his upper chest and face and gazes at them for long periods (A). He can hold things in his hands for quite a while, too (B).

position. He takes swipes with his hands at things he's interested in but usually misses them. He can hold things in one hand or the other for quite a long time if they're placed there, but he can't retrieve them when he drops them, nor can he voluntarily let go of an object. Four-month-olds pay attention to objects and attempt to reach them. A 5-month-old can actually reach for and grasp an object.

The 4- to 5-month-old still has a palmar, or "mitten," grasp, gripping an object in the palm of his hand. Although he can't pick up small objects, he does notice them more than he did before. Whereas it used to take something like a big red ball to catch his attention, now he notices something as tiny as a raisin.

On his tummy, supporting himself on his hands, he can lift both his head and chest off the examining table. He rolls over one way, usually from stomach to back. He can also balance on his tummy and make swimming motions with his arms and legs. Held in a standing position, he can bear some weight on his legs, often with his feet turned out, which is normal. At 5 months of age, babies accept weight

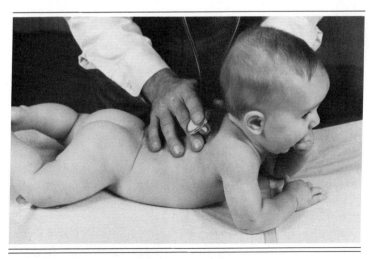

On his tummy a 4-month-old can lift his head and chest well off the examining table.

on their legs without coming up on their toes, also a sign of normal development.

Personal/Social   Socially, he laughs out loud, squeals with delight, and responds with his whole body to things that please him. He waves his arms, kicks his legs, and pants with pleasure. He recognizes familiar faces and enjoys being with other family members where there is noise and activity.

Language/Communication   At age 4 months, babies laugh out loud and squeal in response to social situations. They also "talk" to their toys, their parents, and their brothers and sisters. In an effort to communicate with others, they don't wait to be noticed or spoken to. Rather, they take the initiative by vocalizing and smiling at the person whose attention they want. At 5 months they can tell the difference between their own family and strangers.

Measuring Development   Your baby's doctor keeps careful track of his development. She tests some developmental milestones during the well baby checkup and asks about others. Questions at the 4- to 5-months checkup will probably include "Is he rolling over yet? Does he vocalize or try to talk? Does he turn his head towards sounds?" In addition, there are tests that can help show whether or not a child is developing normally. Although professional evaluation is available, it's important to remember that there is an astonishingly wide range of what can be considered "normal" development. For example, some perfectly normal babies walk as early as 9 months, others not until 16 months. And although most babies fall somewhere between these two "norms," a few normal babies walk even earlier and later than that.

It's also important to point out that development doesn't occur in a steady, straight line. Plotted on a graph, a baby's development would look more like a spiral. There could be lulls in development when babies seem to stop for a breather on one plateau before pushing forward to the next. Sometimes illness accounts for these lulls. At other times they occur because one aspect of development becomes so intense that another falls behind. A baby working hard on verbal skills may fall behind on motor skills temporarily. Such lulls or delays are frequently normal and do not necessarily require instant professional evaluation.

One of the most popular screening devices in the United States is the Denver Developmental Screening Test (DDST). The DDST was devised by studying the developmental progress of more than 1,000 normal children from ages 2 weeks to 6 years, all residents of Denver, Colorado. The test is administered by trained examiners who supervise children in a number of developmental tasks, simple ones for newborns, more complex ones for older children. A newborn who kicks both legs and waves both arms with equal vigor is automatically given a "pass" in the fine motor category. Other newborn tasks include looking at the examiner's face when spoken to and responding to the sound of a bell rung softly near one ear. Older children are instructed to do things like jump with both feet, kick a ball forward, and build a tower of cubes. Tasks are categorized as gross motor (head control, sitting, standing, walking, and so on), language (making noises, laughing, talking, and so on), fine motor—adaptive (eye and hand coordination), and personal—social (smiling, playing, imitating household chores).

Each development—smiling, walking, talking—is illustrated on a scoring sheet by a bar that shows at what age each test item was performed by 25 percent, 50 percent, 75 percent, and 90 percent of the Denver children tested. The DDST shows, for example, that 25 percent of children play pat-a-cake at 7 months, 50 percent play it by 9 months, and 75 percent by 9 months and 3 weeks. By age 13 months, 95 percent of the children tested played pat-a-cake. The range of normal for this task, then, is wide—7 months to 13 months—as it is for most tasks. Failing a task often means no more than that the examiner will note the child's failure and test the item again at a future date. Investigating the child further immediately isn't necessarily indicated.

The DDST is not an IQ test. It is not even usually performed routinely by pediatricians in their private practices. In some other clinical settings, such as university hospital pediatric clinics, it is sometimes routinely performed. Often this is to give students practice in administering it, not necessarily because developmental delays are suspected.

There is no universal agreement about the time frames of developmental milestones. Dr. Ronald Illingworth, a British pediatrician, points out that the DDST percentiles disagree with another study, the Newcastle, that measured some of the same milestones. The Newcastle study, for example, showed that 97 percent of children studied could walk alone by age 19.4 months, whereas the Denver scale shows 14.3 months for the same task. Illingworth agrees with neither. He has seen dozens of children unable to walk alone later than indicated as normal by either study. He believes further that the percentile distribution of developmental milestones is of little value in the first place and that it is probably never possible to draw a clear-cut line between normal and abnormal.

Nonetheless, it is useful for parents to know that there are assessment devices currently in use. In addition to the DDST, there are the Bayley Infant Scale, the Brazelton Neonatal Behavioral Assessment Scale, and the Milani–Comparetti Motor Development Screening Test. Also, Doctors Arnold Gesell and Catherine Amatruda developed an examination for determining developmental and neurological progress.

Although there is disagreement about the ages at which children normally perform various tasks, it is agreed that there is a wide range of normal. It is also true that parents who think their children are slow to do things worry and look for reassurance. Sometimes a screening test can provide that reassurance. It can teach patience to parents who may be in a hurry to have their baby keep up with the baby next door.

NUTRITION

Solids, semisolids actually, will probably be discussed today. Also, iron, vitamins, and fluoride will likely be added to the baby's diet if they haven't already been added. At 4 months of age your baby is finally physically ready for solid foods. He has good head control. When he sits up, his head no longer bobs up and down. That means his mouth is no longer a moving target for a spoonful of food. His tongue, lips, and jaws, which have moved as a single, sucking unit in the past, are now ready to work independently, as they must in order to handle solids. He still can't really chew for another two months or so, though. A more important sign of readiness for solids is that your baby has probably begun to express an interest in the food he sees other family members eating. He may even have begun to take swipes at table food.

Solid food is given at 4 months more for the experience than for its nutrient value. The baby is still getting all the nutrients he needs from milk. Although solids aren't necessary, though, now is a good time to get your baby accustomed to them. He is more receptive to new tastes and textures than he will be when he's older. But, although babies are normally quite accepting of new foods at this age and are ready physically in many ways, too, they are still susceptible to developing food allergies and intolerances because of the relative immaturity of their gastrointestinal (GI) tracts. At 4 months the GI tract is still not fully ready to take on the foreign proteins in solid food, so your doctor will have you go slowly with new foods and watch for food allergies, which can be a serious problem for some babies.

Most parents know that food allergies can cause hives or a skin rash called eczema, but few realize that the problems can be much more than skin deep. The GI system can also be upset, causing nausea, vomiting, and diarrhea. The respiratory system can be affected, with coughing, wheezing, runny nose, and even ear complications. Food allergy commonly causes serous otitis media, an accumulation of fluid in the child's middle ear. Sometimes, though rarely, babies have a systemic reaction, meaning that every part of their body is affected. A reaction can take place in minutes, hours, days or weeks from the time the offending food has been eaten by the baby. That's why it's best to introduce only one new food at a time and watch the baby closely for any adverse reactions.

Foods that cause a problem must be eliminated from the baby's diet and reintroduced later under the doctor's supervision. Whole milk and milk products, eggs—especially egg whites—and wheat are considered to be highly allergenic for babies and are traditionally withheld from the diet until age 6 months, 9 months, or even a year.

If you will be feeding your baby semisolid foods sometime between this checkup and the next, watch for the following signs of food intolerance or allergy so that they can be reported to the doctor's office.

- Vomiting
- Diarrhea
- Runny nose
- Coughing or wheezing
- Rash

There are four food groups: milk and milk products, meats, breads and cereals, and fruits and vegetables. It is customary to start babies on solids with a single-grain cereal. Iron-fortified rice is usually chosen because of its relative freedom from producing allergy. If you were to start instead with a mixed cereal of, say, barley and oats, and the baby developed an allergy, you wouldn't know which of the two grains was responsible. And by feeding the grains to the baby again, one at a time, to identify the problem, you would have to make the baby sick again.

In the beginning babies are most accepting of foods that have a thin consistency, so the rice cereal should be thinned out considerably with formula. When orange juice is introduced into the baby's diet at about age 6 months, it can be used to mix the cereal. There is evidence that orange juice and other vitamin-C-fortified fruit juices actually enhance iron absorption. At first, only a tablespoonful or two of cereal should be offered once a day. The time of day isn't important, but it should be a time when the baby is hungry because then he will be more willing to accept it.

Increase the amount gradually over a period of about a week to three or four tablespoons per feeding.

Use a spoon that is small enough for the baby's mouth, and be prepared for some of the cereal to come right back out at first. This isn't because he doesn't like it, but because he is mouthing it as he would milk. He pushes his mouth, jaws, and tongue forward in a sucking motion (called the extrusion reflex) that causes some of the cereal to be swallowed, some to stay in his mouth, and some to come dribbling back down his chin. He'll do better with practice and as his jaw and tongue develop independent motion.

After a week of success with rice cereal, try something else for another week. By introducing new foods one at a time, it is easier to identify the cause of any problems that develop. Look for allergy or intolerance with each new food you introduce. Signs, again, are vomiting, diarrhea, rash, hives, coughing, wheezing, runny nose, ear infection, and rarely shock.

Traditionally, strained fruits and fruit juices (not citrus) are introduced after cereal. Fruits provide carbohydrates, vitamins, minerals, and fiber. Because they are naturally high in sugar and calories, sugar should not be added. Most babies like bananas, and these can easily be strained or mashed at home. Fruit juice may be offered in a cup, a few ounces at a time. Some nutritionists believe that juice should not be offered in a bottle because it becomes a kind of pacifier.

Introduce strained vegetables into the baby's diet next, at about age 5 months. Give him yellow ones first—because they cause fewer allergies—then green. Vegetables have the fewest calories per unit of volume and provide a good deal of fiber.

Meats are usually introduced last. In fact, the doctor may not want you to start them until after the next checkup at 6 months. Because commercially prepared strained meats stick to the roof of a baby's mouth like a bolux of peanut butter, they may not be as well received as some of the other tastes he's been enjoying. Try diluting them with a little tap water. Of all the food groups, meat is the highest in protein. Meats also contain iron and vitamins. Because they cause fewer allergies, lamb and veal are usually introduced first, then beef and pork.

Home-Prepared Food   You can easily prepare food for your baby at home, but the food should be especially for the baby. Table scraps, salted in the cooking and again at the table, aren't good for him. The food should be prepared on a clean surface to prevent bacterial contamination, then placed into ice-cube trays and stored in the freezer until needed. One defrosted cube makes a single serving for baby. To strain food, you can use a fancy food processor, a blender, or the old-fashioned, time-tested (and *cheap*) way of forcing the food through a strainer with a spoon.

Vegetables should be fresh or frozen but not canned. Canned vegetables and soups contain excessive amounts of sodium chloride (salt) as well as a flavor enhancer called monosodium glutamate that is also very high in salt. Salt has been implicated as a cause of high blood pressure (hypertension), which affects 20 percent or more of adult Americans. It makes good sense to reduce salt intake in infants as a preventive measure against this disease, which, in turn, is a leading factor in stroke and heart disease.

Beets, carrots, and spinach are considered to be un-safe for babies less than 4 months old, and some doctors withhold them until age 6 months for good measure. This is because they may cause methemoglobinemia, a serious disease that affects red blood cells so that they can no longer transport oxygen properly through the body. Cucumbers, onions, cabbage, and broccoli are considered hard to digest and are usually withheld until the baby is older.

Commercial Baby Foods   Although they are gener-ally more expensive than foods you prepare yourself, strained commercial baby foods are acceptable and pro-vide a wide variety from which to choose. There are at least 100 varieties of baby foods on store shelves, but it isn't necessary for the baby to become a gourmet. A jar should be opened, stored properly, and finished before opening another jar. Otherwise the refrigerator would be filled with half-empty jars and spoilage would be a problem. Gerber, Heinz, and Beech-Nut baby foods are packed with a pop-top lid for reasons of health. When you buy the foods, you can run your finger over the lid to be sure the button is slightly indented and not already popped. Then, when you get the food home and open the jar, the small button in the center of the lid should pop up. This tells you that the seal hasn't been broken before and that the food inside is safe from harmful bacteria.

Opened jars of fruits and fruit juices should keep in the refrigerator without spoiling for 72 hours. Other foods may be stored safely for 48 hours, provided that you've removed the desired amount of food at each feeding, then promptly recapped the jar and refrigerated the rest. If you feed the baby directly from the jar, bacteria from his mouth will contaminate the food and its safety can no longer be guaranteed.

Most commercial baby foods no longer contain any food additives, although they did until fairly recently. Lucky baby. As adults we have become unwilling food-additive junkies. There are about 3,000 food additives on the market today—sweeteners, preservatives, salts, bleaches, and a host of artificial colors and flavors (1,610 artificial and 50 natural flavors alone!). Trying to avoid them is a lot like trying to keep dry in a rainstorm by dancing between the raindrops.

The labels on baby food jars assure you that no sugar, salt, or anything else has been added—except sometimes vitamins and minerals. And occasionally you will notice that either rice cereal or cornstarch have been added. This is to preserve the shelf life of the product by preventing it from separating in the jar and looking unappetizing. Become a reader of labels. Many baby food jars have the complete story of their contents, including calories, right there on the label. Calories count for babies just as they do for the rest of us, so it's crucial that you be aware that some baby foods are higher in calories than others. Fruit is fruit and meat is meat, but the calories may surprise you. Gerber's strained peas in a 4½-ounce jar contains 60 calories, for example, whereas the same size jar of green beans contains only 40. Strained beef clocks in with a sedate 89 calories, but strained chicken packs 134, almost 50 percent more! Some baby foods don't show caloric content on the label. In this case you can write the manufacturer for information about the foods they produce. See the resources section at the end of this chapter for names and addresses.

Keep in mind that some baby foods have been designed to appeal to adult tastes and to draw the attention of an adult shopper. Products like peach cobbler and dutch apple dessert were not so much concocted to appeal to baby as to Mom and Dad. To a baby a peach is a peach and an apple an apple.

Special Diets   Vegetarianism, vegan diets, Zen macrobiotics, and megavitamin therapy have become part of the American way of life. A modified vegetarian diet that permits milk and dairy products is a healthy enough one for an infant and growing child. Although there is no meat in the diet, sufficient milk and eggs can provide enough protein for a healthy, well-balanced diet.

Pure vegetarian and vegan diets are somewhat trickier, because a diet that is purely vegetable can be so high in bulk that it may not contain the minimum number of calories required for growth. By carefully combining certain vegetables and cereals, a satisfactory level of protein can be achieved, however. Supplements of vitamin B12 are almost always needed eventually in such a diet.

The Zen macrobiotic diet is considered dangerous for babies by both nutritionists and pediatricians alike. There is evidence that the Zen macrobiotic food mixture for babies as it is presently available is insufficient to sustain normal growth and development in the first year of life. Similarly, megavitamin practices—taking more than 10 times the recommended daily dose of various vitamins—can be extremely dangerous for babies and young children, as discussed in Chapter 5, "The 2–4 Weeks Checkup."

Please understand that doctors are not interested in interfering with your lifestyle. In fact, it is very difficult for health professionals to know how to approach parents who maintain alternative diets. Doctors are only interested in the health and normal development of the babies in their care. There is a critical growth period in a baby's life that can easily be interrupted and altered by insufficient nutrition. The harm done can never be corrected.

Don't overfeed your baby. A fat baby isn't necessarily a healthy baby, and it takes only a few too many calories per day to produce a youngster who begins to resemble a Christmas goose. Given a chance, babies will not normally eat more than they need for their own growth and health. They even signal when they're full. They turn away, or shut their mouths, or start to cry, or even fall asleep. That's your cue to quit feeding them. Of course, occasionally you're blessed with a little gourmand who would eat until he threw up if you let him, but babies like that are unusual. It is, however, normal and healthy for babies to be a bit on the chubby side. Most of the first year of life is a time to lay down fat tissue in reasonable amounts. Later in the first year the emphasis changes to the production of muscle, and the child undergoes a normal dropoff in appetite.

Unfortunately, babies can be trained to link food with emotion instead of hunger. If something "good" is stuffed into their mouths every time they cry, if snacking and cleaning their plates at every meal become a way of life, they get fat just like the rest of us. Overfeeding a baby can increase the number of fat cells he produces, a factor that contributes to his being an obese adult. We know that once the body creates a fat cell, it's a fat cell forever, so it's important that you not train your baby to confuse eating with emotional gratification. That doesn't mean, of course, that you shouldn't make every mealtime as pleasant as possible. You should. Meals are important social events for babies and grownups alike.

PARENT CONCERNS

(These are only some of the concerns parents have at this checkup. Be sure you have yours written down to discuss with the doctor.)

Drooling   Don't worry about drooling. It may or may not have to do with teething. Although most babies don't get their first tooth until age 5 or 6 months or even later, excessive drooling can sometimes precede that event by many weeks. Also, babies drool even when they aren't teething. Until they do have teeth to form a kind of dam across their lower jaw, there isn't anything to keep the saliva back and encourage them to swallow their own spit. They're perfectly happy to have it dribbling down their chins. The only problem it can cause is a patch of dry skin on the lower chin where saliva runs constantly.

Sleep Patterns   Normally 4- to 5-month old babies sleep through the night, 10 to 12 hours without crying. If your baby is not doing so, he probably will in another month or so. From now on his sleep patterns will change very little. A one-year-old, for example, is awake for only an hour a day more than a 2-month-old. In the first year the number of naps decreases, though, from three to two.

Thumbsucking   It is 100 percent normal for babies to suck their thumbs or fingers. Sucking is their primary survival reflex, which very soon becomes associated with gratification and pleasure as well. Little wonder, then, that they discover their own thumbs as a source of gratification and as a means to release tension and anxiety before sleep. Some infants seem to be born with knowledge of the pleasures of thumbsucking. They enter the world with thumbs that appear to be wet, wrinkled, and already well sucked.

Thumbsucking usually self-corrects—along with nudging from parents and peers—some time after age 4 years. It becomes a concern at age 5 or 6, when jawbones are permanently fusing. It is not uncommon, however, for the habit to persist well into preteenage years, where it may finally be dealt with by an orthodontist before he begins his work.

REMINDERS

Safety Topics   Car seats, baby equipment, rolling over, danger from swallowing small objects. See Chapter 3.

Upper Respiratory Tract Infections (URIs)   From now on, you should be on the lookout for URIs (coughs, colds, and sore throats). They begin in the first year of life and continue with some frequency until age 6 or 7 years. During that entire period the average child has anywhere from three to six colds each year.

URIs are usually, but not always, caused by viruses. A single virus in one family may produce a different illness in each family member. Mom may respond with a head cold, Dad with a cough and sore throat, and baby with croup—all from the same virus.

Babies can't be protected very well against URIs, and in any case they need to build up as much immunity as they can as soon as possible, so there are really no special precautions you can take. Symptoms may include runny nose, stuffiness, and cough.

Don't assume you can treat your baby's cold yourself. Although it is okay for grownups to treat their own colds, a URI in a baby should be brought to the attention of a doctor. Cough syrup, for example, a nonprescription item for everybody else in the family, must be prescribed by a physician for a child less than 3 years of age.

At this checkup your doctor may suggest that you buy a small-bulb syringe, just in case. It is used to *gently* suction mucus from the baby's nose, which must be kept clear at all times. (You may remember that young babies are able to breathe only through their noses.) Vaporizers for the nursery are useful when a URI includes coughing and chest congestion, but only cold-air models are recommended. Hot-steam vaporizers are dangerous.

Sometimes URIs become chronic (linger at a low level with the child's never being quite well). In those cases the child may need to be checked further. URIs also include ear infections, and they too can become chronic. Ear infections are discussed in Chapter 9.

Toys   Rattles, suction toys for high-chair trays.

NEXT CHECKUP

Your baby's next checkup will be in two months, when he is 6 or 7 months old. Call the doctor before then, of course, if there are any problems. In the meantime, be looking for the following milestones in development which will appear soon, perhaps before the next checkup.

- Rolls over both ways
- Sits by self
- Transfers objects from hand to hand
- Becomes fearful of strangers

How you truly feel about your baby continues to be important. Do you think he fits well into the family situation? Is he the kind of child you were expecting? Can you cope with and relate to him? If your answer is "no" to any of these questions, talk to your doctor about it. Your negative feelings are not bad or even unusual, but you may need help in finding positive ways to deal with them.

RESOURCES

Beech-Nut Foods   has complete information on the labels about ingredients; additives (usually none); consistency (strained or junior); net weight; and nutrition information—serving size; number of calories; percentage of U.S. Recommended Daily Allowance (RDA) for protein, vitamins, and minerals. A U on the label indicates the contents are kosher.

In addition, there is a national toll-free nutrition hotline that answers Monday through Friday from 9 A.M. to 4 P.M. Eastern time. The telephone number is 1-800-523-6633. In Pennsylvania, call 1-800-492-2384. The Beech-Nut Hotline accepts questions about infant feeding, growth, and behavior. Callers either hear tapes recorded by nutrition experts or have their questions answered by hotline operators using reference books from the Beech-Nut library.

For more product information, send for *A Guide to the Nutritive Values and Ingredients of Beech-Nut Baby Foods,* Beech-Nut, P.O. Box 127, Fort Washington, Pennsylvania 19034.

Gerber Products Company provides complete content information on the labels of its baby foods. In addition, the nutrient values of all Gerber baby foods are available by writing the Professional Communications Department, Gerber Products Company, 445 State Street, Fremont, Michigan 49412. Information comes in a packet entitled *Nutrient Values, Gerber Baby Foods.* The company also attempts to answer written inquiries concerning nutrition.

H. J. Heinz Company Like Gerber and Beech-Nut, Heinz baby foods have pop-top safety lids with clear instructions not to buy the product if the button has already popped up. The lids also show an expiration date for product safety. Heinz baby foods are classified according to the four basic food groups: milk/dairy, vegetable/fruit, meat, and bread/cereal. There are label codes that indicate nonallergy-causing ingredients.

Heinz offers publications for parents. For further information, write to Consumer Relations Department, H. J. Heinz Company, P.O. Box 57, Pittsburgh, Pennsylvania 15230.

Vegetarian Diets *Laurel's Kitchen: A Handbook for Vegetarian Cookery and Nutrition,* by L. Robertson, C. Flinders, and B. Godfrey, Berkeley: Nilgiri Press, 1976, contains recipes for young children and nursing mothers.

Home-Prepared Food: *The Complete New Guide to Preparing Baby Foods* by Sue Castle, Garden City: Doubleday, 1981, is a comprehensive reference. Many other baby food cookbooks are available in bookstores.

8
THE 6–7 MONTHS CHECKUP

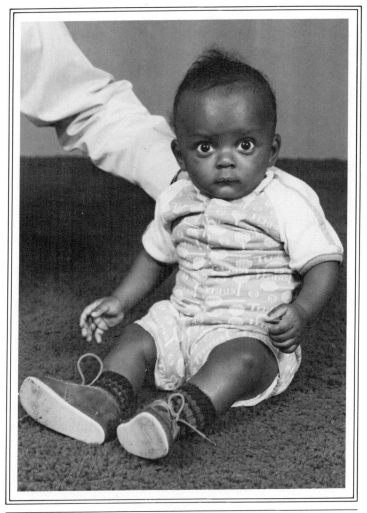

✓ CHECKLIST

6-7 MONTHS CHECKUP

Date _____

Procedures

_____ Weigh and measure   Weight _____

Percentile _____

Height _____

Percentile _____

Head circumference _____

_____ Discuss weight and height gains on growth charts with parents

_____ Immunizations _____ DPT (diphtheria/tetanus/
pertussis) #3

_____ TOPV (oral polio
vaccine) #3 (optional)

_____ Hematocrit (Hct)/Hemoglobin (Hgb) blood test

_____ Cover test of eyes (optional)

_____ Discuss nutrition

_____ Ask about parent concerns

_____ Counsel on safety

PHYSICAL EXAMINATION*

Special attention to:

_____ Hearing (turns quickly toward sound)

_____ Vision (follows a dropped object)

_____ Milestones in development
(rolls over, sits up, bears weight on legs)

*The complete physical examination is described and illustrated in Chapter 4.

The 6- or 7-month-old is usually cooperative and easy for the doctor to examine, although a few babies at that age are stranger-shy and fearful of the doctor. If so, some examination maneuvers may have to be performed with the baby in your lap rather than on the examining table. It is usually just as easy for the doctor either way.

At this visit the baby will be given his third DTP injection, combined toxins and antigens against diphtheria, tetanus (lockjaw), and pertussis (whooping cough). He will probably also get a third dose of oral polio vaccine (TOPV). Although it is considered optional by the American Academy of Pediatrics, a third dose of TOPV is frequently given along with the third DTP injection, particularly to breast-fed babies, in whom polio vaccine may not be as effective, and to babies who live in geographic locations where polio has been a problem in the past.

If your baby hasn't experienced a serious reaction to the previous shots at ages 2 and 4 months, he can reasonably be expected not to have much trouble with these either. There will be no more shots until he is 15 months old, when he will be immunized against measles, mumps, and rubella (German measles). Now that the DTP series is complete, it will provide a high degree of immunity for your baby. To ensure continuing protection, however, booster doses will be necessary periodically for the rest of his life. The first DTP booster will be given when he is 18 months old. The next will be given when he is 4 to 6 years old. Be sure to add this immunization to the permanent records provided at the back of this book.

A hematocrit (Hct) or hemoglobin (Hgb) may be performed at this visit if one or the other hasn't been done previously. The Hct is a blood test to determine the percentage of red blood cells in the baby's blood and to check for iron deficiency anemia, which can be a problem for some babies after age 4 months.

A small sample of blood is taken from the baby's heel and sent to the laboratory, where it is placed in a centrifuge and spun for a few minutes. The spinning separates the blood into two layers, red blood cells at the bottom and yellowish plasma at the top. The Hct represents the percentage of blood that is made up of red blood cells. At age 6 or 7 months, 33 to 42 percent of the baby's blood should consist of red blood cells. A hemoglobin (Hgb) is a chemical test that is sometimes used instead of the Hct to detect anemia.

Different doctors have different schedules for the Hct/ Hgb tests. Sometimes it is done as early as 4 months or as late as 9 months or a year, but it is almost always done at some time in the first year of life. It may be done at any age, of course, if the doctor suspects a problem. Iron deficiency is more common in twins, premature babies, or babies born with obstetrical complications such as placenta previa. Normal, full-term babies are usually born with enough iron stores to last about four months.

Another test that may be performed at this checkup is the cover test, a simple maneuver to check out any nerve or muscle problems with the baby's eyes. The doctor is looking (screening) for crossed eyes, known medically as strabismus or squint. Sometimes a child's eyes cross or wander only when he is tired, a condition called lazy eyes. The cover test involves covering and uncovering each of the child's eyes in turn, usually with a hand. A child with normal eyesight will keep both eyes looking at you even when one eye is covered. When you take your hand away, the eye is looking straight at you. If there is a nerve or muscle problem, however, the eye will wander off as soon as it's covered. Uncovered, it's looking somewhere else. With this simple test the doctor can identify a problem and even tell whether it is a nerve or a muscular one.

Just as the front-end alignment of an automobile must be almost perfect in order for the car to drive well, a child's eyes must be lined up properly in order for him to have normal vision. Eye alignment affects depth perception and the ability to receive images in both eyes and fuse them into a single, integrated picture.

THE PHYSICAL EXAMINATION

Testing for hearing is aided at this checkup by the fact that the normal 6- or 7-month-old turns his head quickly toward the sounds he hears. Although that doesn't necessarily mean his hearing is perfect, it does mean that he can hear test sounds such as the snapping of fingers, clapping of hands, or ringing of a bell that take place out of his line of vision. The examiner usually steps to the side or behind the baby for this test.

This is a test that parents can easily perform at home to check their baby's hearing. Remember, though, that babies eventually habituate to sound. That is, they become accustomed to the sound and stop responding to it.

In testing vision there are two useful devices to assess the visual development that should have occurred since the last checkup. Like the hearing tests, both can easily be done by parents at home. One is to catch the baby's attention with a bright object, such as a pompom of yarn, and then drop the object onto the floor. The baby should look down quickly to see where the pompom has gone. Another indication of normal vision is the baby's new interest in small objects, something that began to develop at age 4 months. He should be able to pay attention to a raisin or pellet placed in front of him and show enough interest to rake at it with his hands. A normal 6-month-old is fully able to focus and fixate with his eyes.

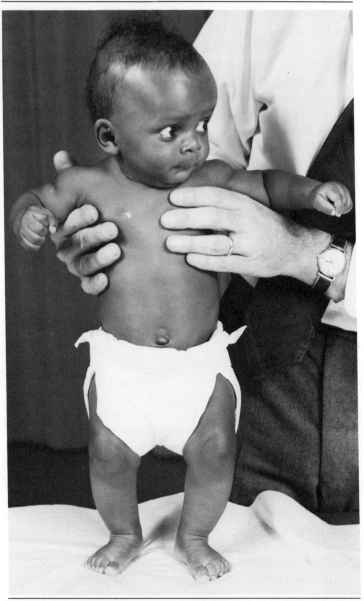

*In a standing position the 6-month old
can bear his full weight on his legs.*

Not all examiners test for vision and hearing at each checkup. Sometimes they just ask "Does the baby seem to hear?" or "Does the baby seem to see?"

Head control will be tested for about the last time at this checkup. When a 6-month-old is pulled to a sitting position from his back, not only is there no head lag, but his head should actually lead his body in anticipation of the movement. He "assists" the doctor with his head as he is pulled to sit. By the time he reaches a sitting position, his chin is all tucked in. Head control is so good that he may even lift his head off the examining table to have a look around when he's lying there on his back.

In a standing position, the 6- or 7-month-old should be able to bear his full weight on his legs, although he may still tend to stand on his toes, which is normal. He no longer keeps his legs locked at the knees, though. Instead, he alternately flexes them and straightens them again so that he bounces when held.

During the physical examination, the doctor will probably abduct the hips to check for hip dislocation. Some doctors believe that if no congenital dislocation has shown up by now, it probably will not, and that hip abduction is not particularly useful beyond this checkup. Other doctors believe the maneuver should be continued throughout the first two years of life.

At this visit, when the doctor opens your baby's mouth, inserts a tongue depressor, and looks inside with a penlight, there may be something to examine besides the soft structures, palate, gums, and tonsils. Teeth. Two bottom central incisors may have erupted by now, although tooth development is extremely variable and not all babies have teeth at age 6 months.

Called primary or deciduous, a baby's first teeth begin to form before he is born. Calcification, the formation of calcium for the teeth that your baby has at 6 months, took place in his jaw during the fifth fetal month. Calcification for the secondary, permanent teeth began at birth and will continue through the first two years of life and beyond.

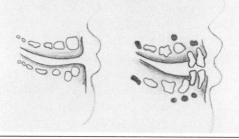

*A baby's first teeth form in his jaw before he
is born (left). Even as his primary teeth are erupting
(right) at age 6 to 9 months, the permanent teeth
that will replace them are forming. Primary teeth are
shown in white, second teeth in black.*

Even as your baby's first teeth are erupting, the permanent
teeth that will replace them are forming.

As soon as your baby has teeth, even if it's only one or
two of them, you may clean them regularly if you choose.
Wherever there are teeth—even if only one or two—there is
an opportunity for infection and decay. The plaque that
forms constantly on teeth may be harmful if it isn't cleaned
off at least once in every 24-hour period. When a baby is
young—6 months to a year—his teeth may be cleaned
once a day, preferably at bedtime. This can be done easily
by wiping the tooth or teeth carefully with a washcloth or
clean square of gauze, either wet or dry. The wiping disrupts
the harmful bacteria colony that forms on the teeth.

The doctor will be especially interested in checking
motor development at this age, for your baby can now do
an astonishing number of things. Each developmental
milestone will be checked either by observing the child
directly or by asking you questions. "Does he feed himself a
cracker? Roll over? Both ways? Does he crawl or creep?"
Crawling is defined as moving by pulling oneself up on
hands or elbows and dragging the legs behind, comman-
do-style. Creeping is getting about on all fours.

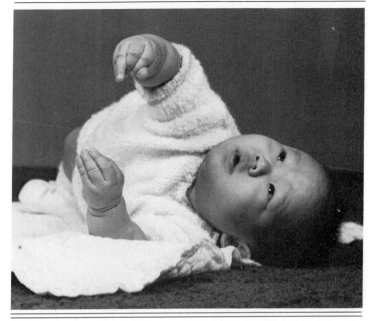

Like most 6-month-olds, Derek can roll over.

MILESTONES IN DEVELOPMENT ± *

Motor/Physical
- Pulled to sit, no head lag
- Sits without support or leaning forward on hands
- On tummy, gets up on all fours
- Crawls
- Rolls over both ways
- Bears weight on legs
- Reaches for object
- Passes object from one hand to other
- Chews

Personal/Social
- Drinks milk from cup

*The plus-or-minus sign indicates that your baby may reach developmental milestones earlier or later than what is indicated here as "average." There is a wide range of normal in child development.

- Holds bottle
- Feeds self cracker
- Smiles spontaneously
- May be anxious about strangers

Language/Communication
- Babbles, imitates sounds

By its very length, this list of developmental milestones shows you how much your baby is progressing. Now, more than ever, you should resist the temptation to compare your 6-month-old with somebody else's. Not every 6-month-old does all of the preceding things "on time," and, as we've noted, there is a very wide range of normal for all developmental milestones. Some normal 6-month-olds crawl and sit unsupported. Others, also perfectly normal, are content to balance on their bellies, flapping their arms and legs, and still need support when they sit.

Your baby is developing at his own rate, according to his unique genetic timetable. If you express concern about your little "flapper" to the doctor, she will probably be able to show you, by means of some skilled maneuvers, that the baby is indeed ready to do all those other things. When he gets around to it.

Motor/Physical   All along, head control has been an important indicator of your baby's motor development because it is the first item of business on the development agenda. From the time he is born, a baby's head is both his biggest body part and his biggest problem. Until he could learn to lift, turn, and in every other way control his head, he couldn't move on to the next stage of development—control of his body. Now that your baby has good control of his head, he is beginning to get body control. When he was an infant and you moved him to a sitting position, his back was very curved. Now when he sits, he may have a nice, straight back. If he sits leaning forward, supporting himself with his arms, however, his back may still be curved.

On his tummy, your baby can bring himself to all fours and has probably developed some kind of mobility, either by crawling, scooting backwards, or rolling. He can prob-

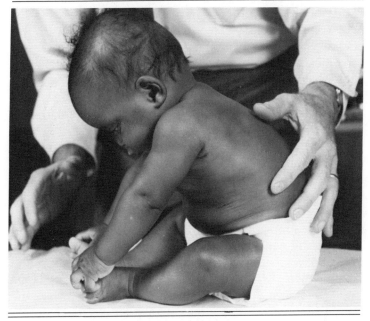

At age 6 months many babies sit leaning forward, supporting themselves with their arms (and sometimes playing with their toes).

ably roll over both ways, the easy way (tummy to back) and the hard way (back to tummy).

In a standing position he can bear a considerable amount of weight on his legs, at the same time keeping his knees flexed (supple, relaxed, and slightly bent). Often he bounces up and down when held in a standing position.

In the area of fine motor development, which involves small muscles and increased eye and hand coordination, your baby is beginning to make some progress, too. He can feed himself a cracker, reach out for something he wants, and work hard to get to a toy that's just out of reach. He may even be able to pass a cube, toy, or other object from one hand to the other, something that usually occurs between the ages of 6 and 8 months. If he is holding an object in one hand and you offer him another object, he may be able to pass the first object to his other hand, accept the new object, and have both hands full at once. But he still can't pick up a tiny object like a pellet or raisin. He lacks the coordination.

The 6-month-old baby still exhibits mostly gross motor activity and skills, that is, skills that involve movement of large muscles and whole limbs. When the baby wants to move his hand, for example, he ends up moving his whole arm. Fine motor skills, those that involve coordination of smaller muscles with the hand and the eye, can only develop when the baby has control of every component of hand movement separately—finger, hand, wrist, lower and upper arm. He doesn't have this control yet because the nerve fibers in his central nervous system have not yet developed myelin, the fatty sheaths that protect and insulate them. The myelin system won't be completed until the nerves have done some more growing. Meanwhile, the baby's motor system is a little bit like an electrical system with a short circuit. The baby tries to move his finger, but his whole arm moves instead.

The 6-month-old is beginning to have a sense of his own body. As a 4-month-old, he regarded his hands intently, but he wasn't quite sure how they got there in front of his face. Now he notices his body parts, particularly his feet, which he captures and plays with on purpose. He may even get a foot into his mouth, which has become an important tool in his learning about objects. It is often said of 6-month-olds that everything goes into their mouths, and it's true. When a baby mouths things, he is actually learning about them—feeling them, biting them, pushing them in and out of his mouth, turning them first one way and then another. Later he will have more sophisticated ways of dealing with objects, but right now it is very normal for him to be exploring them with his mouth. You will need to be sure, of course, that he doesn't get hold of any small objects that could be swallowed or choked on.

A key development at 6 months is that your baby can now chew. The chewing is rudimentary, in that it is done

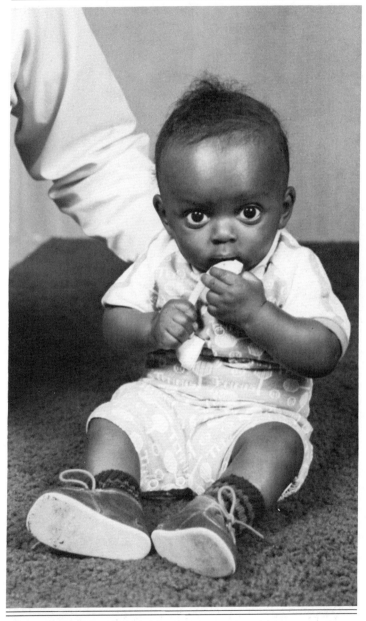

*Everything goes straight
into the mouth of a 6-month-old.*

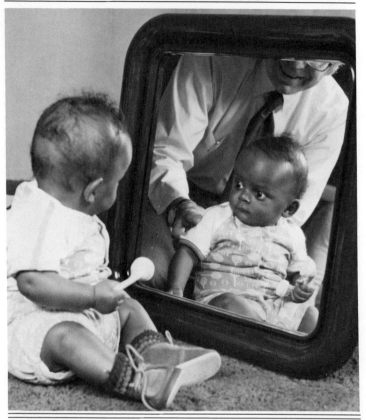

Mirrors are fascinating for babies of all ages.

with a straightforward up-and-down motion of the jaws and lacks the more sophisticated jaw rotation that will develop later. Nonetheless, this new chewing ability is an important landmark for parents to know about and respond to. See "Nutrition," later in this chapter, for details.

Personal/Social At this age your baby will enjoy looking at himself in a mirror. Not only will he be very interested in what he sees, but he'll pat his own image, smile, and have a wonderful time. Six-month-olds smile spontaneously without encouragement and are pleasant socially, although some may begin to show signs of stranger anxiety. Some 6-month-olds are also anxious about being separated from their parents, particularly their mothers, although separation anxiety is perhaps more common in 8-month-olds. Happily, all babies eventually learn that, although Mom and Dad go away, they also come back. Sometimes when babies of 6 to 8 months cry in the middle of the night, it is from separation anxiety. All babies waken regularly during the night from the time of birth, but

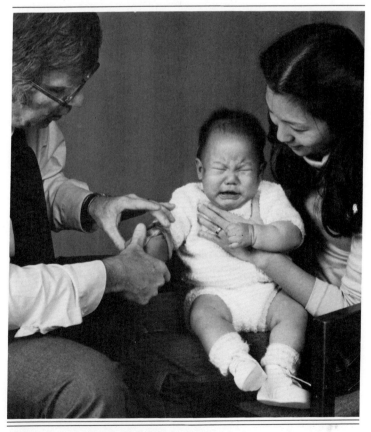

*Stranger anxiety may begin as early as
age 6 months—especially in the doctor's office.*

at age 8 months or so, they begin to feel anxious that their parents aren't there with them. See "Parents Concerns," later in this chapter, for tips on how to handle this.

The 6-month-old can do a number of things for himself. He can hold his own bottle, drink milk or juice from a cup (with help), and feed himself a cracker.

Language/Communication The sounds your baby makes have become more varied. He goes "mmmmmmmmmmm" when he's fussing or complaining. He also tries very hard to imitate the sounds you make, particularly vowel sounds like "aah" and "ooh." This is called echolalia. And if you make a Bronx cheer, or razzing sound, with your mouth, he imitates it joyfully.

NUTRITION

Counseling on nutrition will probably be an important part of this checkup. If you haven't already done so, introduce your baby to solid foods now, for he is really ready for

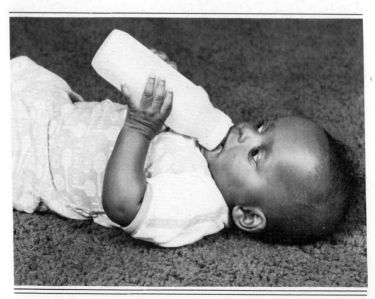

A 6-month-old can hold his own bottle.

them. He can chew, a physical development that usually coincides with his getting a tooth or two. But even if he has no teeth, he can still chew. As a newborn, he could only move his lower jaw forward and back again in unison with his tongue and lips. Jaw, tongue, and lips worked together as a kind of slick sucking machine. Now he can make them work independently to munch and chew. And he needs immediate practice with his chewing.

A baby who isn't given at least some experience with solid foods at age 6 months may have difficulty accepting them later. He doesn't need to eat a lot of solids—his nutritional needs can still be met by milk alone—but he does need the experience of chewing. The doctor may recommend that you feed your baby solids of some kind at least three times a day, to coincide with breakfast, lunch, and dinner. Three meals plus four milk feedings a day are often suggested. Be sure to include all four food groups in his diet—bread and cereals, milk and milk products, fruits and vegetables, and meats.

Now that your 6-month-old can chew, he can also handle small lumps. Among the carefully selected table foods appropriate at this time are applesauce and mashed potatoes as well as baked potatoes, cooked carrots, and bananas that have been mashed with a fork; finely ground beef; and mashed peas.

Your baby will also enjoy finger foods that he can hold in his fist and munch at his own pace. Finger foods introduced at this age might more properly be called fist foods, for your baby doesn't have independent use of his fingers yet. He still has a palmar, or "mitten" grasp, so that he can't let go of things voluntarily. In other words, he'll hold food tightly in his fist until he munches down to his knuckles. So you need to select something that is long enough to stick out at the top of his fist. Cheese cut into strips works well. As he chews down to his fist, you should open his hand and push the food up for him so he can get some more. You can see why a Cheerio would be very frustrating for a child this age. If he managed to get it into his fist at all (very unlikely because of his undeveloped grasp), it would be trapped there. He couldn't even open his hand to see what in the world had happened to it. Save the Cheerios and other dried cereal until he's about 10 months old, when the thumb and forefinger (pincer) grasp begins to develop.

Be careful, too, to avoid splinter foods. These are foods like cookies that break off into small pieces when the baby works at them with his mouth. There is danger of his inhaling and choking on the pieces that splinter off. Commercially prepared arrowroot cookies are a better choice than graham crackers, for example, because graham crackers splinter. Oven-dried toast strips prepared in your own oven are also a good choice.

If you feed your baby commercial baby foods, he is ready now for junior foods rather than strained ones. Although no salt is added in the commercial preparation of strained foods, junior foods are now available from Gerber baby foods with a low-salt option. Check the labels carefully, as always, to be sure you know which you are buying.

Variety is essential in your baby's diet. Even though most of his nutrients will continue to come from milk for a while longer, it's important that he become used to a number of different foods. It will help make him a less picky eater later.

Calories are an important consideration, too. Overfeeding your baby will make him fat, not healthy. When solid foods are added to his diet, milk intake must be reduced. Otherwise he will be getting too many calories. The baby should drink no more than 28 ounces of milk in a 24-hour period. When you're counting calories, remember that milk contains 20 calories per ounce. Cereal contains more calories than that per ounce; meat and vegetables fewer. If your baby were fed cereal three times a day, for example, he would be getting too many calories. If you served him only vegetables, he would get too few.

A typical day's menu for a 6-month-old might look something like this.

Breakfast Iron-fortified rice cereal mixed with milk or vitamin-C-fortified fruit juice, no sugar added. Breast milk or formula.

Midmorning   Orange juice (usually introduced at about this age).

Lunch   Meat. Vegetable (yellow or green). Milk.

Dinner   Meat if not given at lunch. Potato or cereal. Yellow or green vegetable. Fruit. Cottage cheese or yogurt. Milk.

Bedtime   Milk (*not* in a bottle that baby is allowed to fall asleep with).

Introduce new foods one at a time and at least a week apart so that you can identify a troublesome food that causes allergy or intolerance. Details for introducing new foods are discussed in the nutrition section of Chapter 7.

Six months is the earliest possible age that weaning from the breast is recommended because maturation and development of the gastrointestinal tract at 6 months allows it to handle the foreign proteins contained in cow's milk and other foods. Many mothers choose to breast-feed for a longer period, but if you are going to stop breast-feeding now, your baby should be given a commercial formula or evaporated milk formula, not cow's milk. This is because he is still drinking a significant amount of milk a day, and there is evidence that cow's milk in those quantities can cause intestinal bleeding and anemia in some babies. Skim and 2 percent milk are not considered appropriate at this age, either.

Although parents receive this information and counseling from doctors and clinics all over the United States, a discouraging number of parents still wean their babies directly to cow's milk, against the advice of their doctors. The switch to cow's milk can be safely made after the baby is about a year old, when he is taking most of his nourishment from solid foods and his milk intake has been reduced to about 16 ounces a day.

Bedtime bottles should be fed to your baby *before* he is put to bed. The bottles a baby falls asleep with are devastating to his developing teeth. The milk, sugar water, or juice in the bottle pool in his mouth, bathing his teeth in harmful sugar solutions and damaging his teeth even as they break the surface of his gums.

PARENT CONCERNS

(These are only some of the concerns parents have at this checkup. Be sure you have yours written down to discuss with the doctor.)

Night Wakenings   Night wakenings are sometimes a natural part of a baby's separation anxiety. He wakes up at night, finds himself alone, and panics. He cries because he's frightened and anxious about not having you there with him. You can help by giving him a few minutes to work it out for himself. If he doesn't quiet down, you may have to go to his room, pat him, say a few reassuring words, and leave. This is usually enough to calm him without rewarding him to the extent that he would like to make it a nightly social event.

Parent Preference   Sometimes, at about the same time he demonstrates separation and stranger anxiety, a baby begins to show preference for one parent or another. In many families, the baby spends most of his time with his mother, and the preference, therefore, is for her. It helps fathers to know that the rejection is common and temporary.

Shoes   Except for bronzing, there's no reason for a baby to have shoes until he begins to walk. If you do buy shoes for him now, be sure they have soft soles, sufficient growing room, and laces that aren't tied too tightly.

Teething   A teething ring that has been cooled in the refrigerator will feel good on baby's gums. No medication should be applied to the gums. Especially dangerous are the ones with names that end in *-caine.* These contain anesthetic agents that can cause an allergic response. Your doctor may also prescribe aspirin or Tylenol for teething discomfort.

REMINDERS

Safety Topics   Childproofing the house, buying a first aid book, syrup of ipecac, falls, choking, drowning, poisoning, and burns. See Chapter 3.

Pets   Children at this age treat all objects the same.

They explore by poking and pulling. Vigorously. Even the best-natured pet may snap at this kind of treatment. Protect your baby and your pet from each other by making sure the baby doesn't unknowingly hurt the animal.

Toy Boxes Toy boxes with hinged tops are danger-ous because a baby's fingers can become caught in them. Any toy box that has a lid and is big enough for a baby or young child to crawl into should have air holes drilled in it as a safety measure. This will prevent the child's accidentally suffocating.

Toys Suitable toys for this age are mirrors (not glass), stuffed animals, stacking toys, and suction toys for the high chair. Also suitable are household utensils such as measuring cups and spoons. Some messy play is okay—a shallow basin of water with float toys, for example.

NEXT CHECKUP

Your baby's next well baby checkup will probably be in three months, when he is 9 months old, although some doctors wait until age one year, before seeing the baby again. Between now and the next checkup, be looking for the following milestones in development. (See the next chapter for details.)

- Sits well by self
- Creeps on all fours
- Stands holding on
- May cruise (walk holding on to things)
- Begins to develop a pincer grasp with thumb and forefinger (This is an important development because it means he can pick up and swallow small objects, which you must be careful to keep out of his reach.)
- Says "Dada" or "Mama" (but doesn't associate anybody with the words yet)
- Responds to own name
- Plays peek-a-boo (so be ready to play it with him)

9
The 9–10 MONTHS CHECKUP

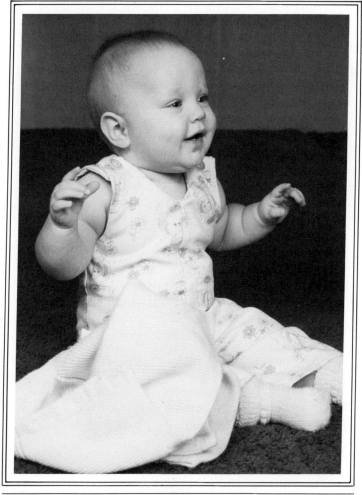

✓ CHECKLIST

9–10 MONTHS CHECKUP

Date _____

Procedures

_____ Weigh and Measure

Weight _____

Percentile _____

Height _____

Percentile _____

Head Circumference _____

_____ Discuss weight and height gains on growth charts with parents

_____ Hematocrit (Hct)/Hemoglobin (Hgb) if not done previously

_____ Tuberculosis test (optional)

_____ Cover test (for crossed eyes) if not done previously

_____ Discuss nutrition

_____ Ask about parent concerns

_____ Counsel on safety

PHYSICAL EXAMINATION*

Special attention to:

_____ Hearing

_____ Vision

_____ Mouth for teeth

_____ Spine, sitting and standing

_____ Developmental milestones (sits, creeps, may cruise)

The complete physical examination is described and illustrated in Chapter 4.

There are no special procedures attached to the 9–10 months checkup, no immunizations—unless they are for catchup—no tests, no change in the weighing and measuring procedures. In fact, some doctors don't even schedule well baby checkups at this age. A checkup at 9 months does, however, provide a good break between the 6–7 months and one-year checkups.

An eye test to check for crossed eyes may be performed at this time if it wasn't done earlier. Called a cover test, it identifies crossed, wandering, and lazy eyes. See Chapter 8 for details. At age 9 months, a baby's eyes should no longer be crossed at any time. If they are, an ophthalmologist should be consulted.

Some doctors test for tuberculosis (TB) at this age in high-risk populations or where there has been a known exposure to the disease. Although TB is not the deadly scourge of mankind that it once was, it still has not been eradicated everywhere, perhaps not even from your own community. The American Academy of Pediatrics (AAP) recommends that TB testing be done at age one year, recognizing that individual doctors must implement the recommendation, depending on circumstances in their own communities. As for repeat testing, the AAP recommends it be done at least once a year and more frequently if local circumstances indicate it.

The simplest but least reliable method of testing is with the TB tine. It is performed by puncturing the baby's lower forearm with a short-pronged tine that has been dipped in a sterile tuberculin preparation. Some health professionals prefer the more reliable method of injecting the preparation directly under the skin with a needle. This is known as the PPD or Mantoux method. There is no risk of getting the disease from either procedure.

The parent is asked to examine the area of the puncture or injection within 48 to 72 hours, depending on the method used. Some doctors and nurses circle the area on the baby's skin with a ballpoint pen to remind parents that a "reading" needs to be done. If the skin becomes red or hard or if a pimple or blister forms at the site, it should be reported to the doctor. If not, as is usually the case, your baby is free of tuberculosis.

Assessing your baby's normal ability to see and hear becomes a little easier as she gets older. When she hears a sound now, she should turn immediately to it. Although this doesn't guarantee that she has a full range of normal hearing, it does indicate that she is able to hear certain sounds that take place out of her line of vision.

Children with impaired hearing do not turn to locate the source of sound. Another clue is that they make no attempt to imitate the sounds their parents make. They don't vocalize as much as do children with normal hearing, and when they do, they tend to repeat the same sound in a dull monotone that lacks the normal, rich variety of sounds that babies should make.

Normal speech development is the most important indication of normal hearing. A baby who speaks clearly and has an average or better-than-average vocabulary for her age is probably a baby who hears well. The 9-month-old is on the verge of a speech "explosion." Between now and age 2 years is a critical period in her language development and one in which you should talk to her constantly, read to her, and name objects for her. It's important now more than ever for you to talk to her and encourage her in her efforts to master words. From this month's simple "Mama," she will, with your help, progress to a vocabulary of about six words (some of them not true words) by the time of her next checkup at age one year. That will explode in the second year to a vocabulary of perhaps too many words to count (a minimum of 50 +) by age 2.

THE PHYSICAL EXAMINATION

It's important for the doctor to get a really good look inside the ears at this checkup because a hearing loss can be caused by repeated or lingering (chronic) ear infections. Between the ages of 6 months and 2 years, ear infection is one of the most common and troublesome of childhood illnesses. It is part of the package known as URIs (upper respiratory infections), which also includes coughs, colds, and sore throats (see Chapter 7). Some children develop an ear infection with every head cold they catch. And since children commonly catch an average of three to six head colds each year, you can see what a problem ear infection can be.

The most severe problems occur when the infection is in the middle ear, the area just behind the eardrum. It is a small space sealed off by the eardrum, its air pressure regulated by the Eustachian tube, which connects to the back of the nose and throat. When the Eustachian tube becomes blocked because of a condition such as a head cold, two problems can develop in the middle ear. One is inflammation, called otitis media. The other is trapped fluid, called serous otitis media. The fluid may be relatively clear or it may be infected by bacteria or a virus.

To further complicate the issue, bacterial infections can be treated with antibiotics, but viral infections cannot. Because there is no practical way for the doctor to take a sample of trapped fluid, treatment of ear infection is based on the most likely infection. Under age 3 years, one or two types of bacteria are usually responsible, so treatment is on the basis of the most likely bacterial cause. A red, bulging eardrum usually means an acute bacterial infection, whereas amber-colored fluid behind a nonbulging, re-tracted (sunken) drum usually means chronic serous otitis media. Middle-ear infections may be acute (newly acquired and severe) or chronic (older, lingering, and somewhat milder).

Another problem with ear infection in babies is that it is extremely hard to diagnose. The baby can't tell you her ears hurt, and in fact some infections don't hurt. Some babies do appear to be ill, however. They pull at their ears, run a temperature, or even develop diarrhea as a result of ear infection. Other signs and symptoms include general irritability and discharge (sometimes bloody) from the ear. In short, ear infection can run the gamut from no symptoms at all to every kind of symptom imaginable.

Although antibiotics are often effective against middle-ear infections, they are not always, and the risk of damage to the baby's middle ear is especially great if infections are frequent or chronic. Scar tissue can form, distorting the sounds a baby hears and causing permanent damage and hearing loss.

Sometimes tubes are inserted in the child's ear (tympanostomy) to help drain the fluid from the middle ear. Although this procedure takes only a few minutes, it must be performed under general anesthesia in a hospital operating room by a specialist. Therefore, it is undertaken only after serious consideration. Although criteria vary from specialist to specialist, the usual conditions for installing ear tubes are that there is serous otitis media for a period of at least four months, along with a documented hearing loss. The tubes cause the baby no discomfort. Later, when the period of chronic or repeated infection is past, the tubes are removed. Sometimes they fall out by themselves.

Both the decision to operate and the operation itself are done by an otoloaryngologist, an ear, nose, and throat (ENT) specialist, after referral from your baby's doctor. If you think your baby has had more than her share of ear infections, ask the doctor if he thinks a visit to an ENT specialist would be worthwhile. If you suspect your child has a hearing problem, you should also mention it to the doctor. There are diagnostic tests that can be done to confirm a hearing loss.

Your baby's eyes have also been observed at each

checkup. They have been examined repeatedly for the red reflex, for pupillary response to light, and for crossed eyes as well (see Chapter 4). None of these maneuvers determines how well she actually sees, however.

Babies and little children can't tell you that they have trouble seeing, but they do signal their problem quite clearly in other ways. They hold objects very close when they want to look at them. Sometimes they shut or cover one eye to see better, or they tilt their heads forward when examining an object. They may pick out only the brightest objects from a group of toys, too. Other clues to eye problems are excessive rubbing or blinking of the eyes or squinting in an attempt to see an object better. Eyes that water a great deal or eyelids that are red and crusted should also be a concern to both parents and doctors. If the eyes themselves are red and bloodshot, the baby may be suffering from conjunctivitis, inflammation of the surface of the eye. If you have noticed any of these signs or tendencies in your baby, report them to your doctor right away.

During the mouth examination, the doctor will check for teeth. As a general rule, the number of teeth a baby will

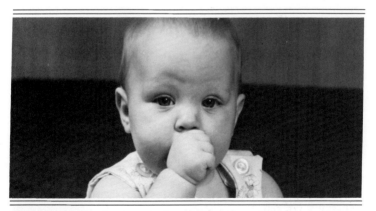

Thumbsucking is a normal activity enjoyed by many babies and young children. It doesn't become a problem until age 5 or 6 years, when bones in the jaw are permanently fusing.

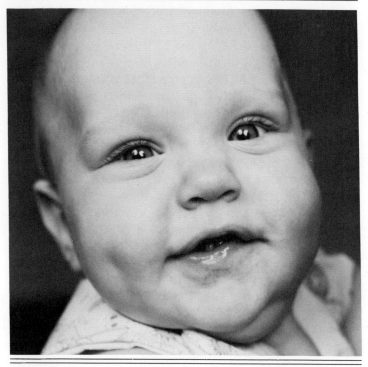

At age 9 months, most babies have two or three teeth. Tooth development is highly variable, however, right up until age 2 years, when there should be a full set of 20.

have at any age in the first 18 months of life is roughly equal to her age in months minus six. By this calculation, a 9-month-old has at least three teeth, and in fact, four teeth—two each on top and bottom center—are not unusual. Next will come the lateral incisors, the teeth on either side of the central incisors. There will be 20 teeth in all. most of them will be in place by the time your baby is 2 years old. Two other general rules are that bottom teeth usually erupt before top teeth and that girls get their teeth slightly earlier than boys.

Diet and general good health are very important to the formation of healthy teeth. Keeping them that way is a matter of careful cleaning, regular dental checkups from age 2 or 3 years on, and continuing sound nutrition and good health. Teeth are pretty wonderful when you stop to think about them. Perfectly designed to tear, cut, grind, and chew every conceivable kind of food, they last a lifetime if given reasonable care.

Although the first 20 baby teeth are only temporary, even they must last five years and longer before their permanent replacements begin to erupt. Care of the first teeth influences the formation of the second teeth. The number-one-enemy of a healthy tooth is sugar. In combination with plaque, the colorless film of bacteria that constantly forms around teeth, it produces an enamel-destroying acid that allows harmful bacteria to penetrate and infect teeth. A tooth that has been so penetrated begins to decay and, without treatment, will eventually be completely destroyed.

Tooth decay is primarily a childhood disease, so parents have to be sugar-smart. Since some researchers and nutritionists think that babies may have a natural sweet preference, your job of keeping sweets under control is sure to be a challenging one. It isn't possible or even advisable, of course, to remove every grain of sugar from the diet. The lactose in baby's milk is a form of sugar. So is the fructose in fruits. Both are a healthy, necessary part of your baby's diet when taken in balance with other foods. Further, when these natural sugars are eaten at mealtimes, their potential harm to teeth is neutralized by other foods and liquids taken at the same meal.

The real culprit is sucrose and refined sugars, the kind found in soft drinks, candy, cookies, and other sweets. Not only is the sugar in these sweets much more highly concentrated, but it does more harm because the sweets are usually eaten between meals, when there are no other foods present to counteract the sugar. So, for good nutrition and for the sake of their teeth, babies should be given low-sugar snacks such as bananas and other fruits, oven-dried toast, dried cereal with no sugar, and cheese.

If your baby has a lot of discomfort when she is

teething, give her something blunt to chew on, such as a rubber teething ring. You may also give her a painkiller (analgesic) like aspirin or Tylenol if your doctor prescribes it. *Do not apply numbing applications directly to her gums, as they are highly allergenic.* You can recognize them by the fact that they frequently have brand names that end in *-caine.*

During the examination the doctor may also be interested in your baby's spine in both the sitting and standing positions. Primarily he is concerned that it is straight and that the baby's posture, sitting and standing, is also straight. Healthy babies have naturally good posture and don't have to be nagged about slumping for many years to come.

When standing, the baby's feet at this age are very flat and seem to have no arch at all. This is normal and doesn't

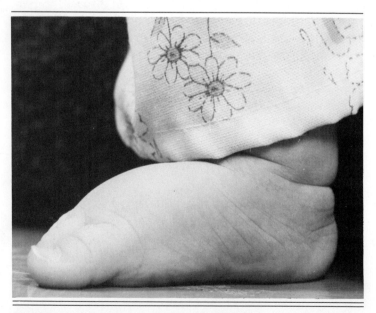

The feet of a 9-month-old are normally very flat and seem to have no arch. This is caused by a fat pad which later disappears.

mean the child is necessarily permanently flat-footed. It is normal, too, for 9-month-olds to stand on their toes and to point their feet out.

Along with these physical findings the doctor will also be interested in the baby's developmental milestones and will probably also spend some time on the subject of nutrition at this visit.

MILESTONES IN DEVELOPMENT ± *

Motor/Physical
- Gets into sitting position by self
- Sits well without support
- Moves from sitting to tummy easily
- Creeps
- May pull self to stand
- Stands holding on
- May cruise (walk sideways, holding on to furniture)
- Uses index finger to approach objects
- Has a thumb-finger (pincer) grasp
- Begins to let go of objects voluntarily

Social/Personal
- Shy with strangers
- Plays pat-a-cake
- Waves bye-bye

Language/Communication
- Says "Dada, Mama"
- May have one other "word"
- Responds to own name

At this checkup it's especially important to remember the plus-or-minus sign that means "maybe sooner, maybe later." This is because so many skills appear or mature between the ninth and tenth months. Take *Mama, Dada,* for instance. The 9-month-old who says these words (and about 75 percent of babies at this age do) doesn't associate anybody in particular with them. They're just sounds that

*The plus-or-minus sign indicates that your baby may reach developmental milestones earlier or later than what is indicated here as "average." There is a wide range of normal in child development.

seem to make the parents happy. By age 10 months, though, she begins to associate the people with the words. Similarly, the typical 9-month-old can only poke at things with her index finger, but at 10 months she can use thumb and forefinger, the beginning of a neat pincer grasp.

Physical Development   The 9-month-old is impressive from the standpoint of motor development. While it took her about six months to get control of her head, it has taken her only half that time to get her trunk under control. She sits without support and with a straight back. She may even get in and out of a sitting position easily by herself, a task that 80 percent of babies can do at age 10 months. In any case, moving from sitting to tummy is easy for her. She also creeps on all fours.

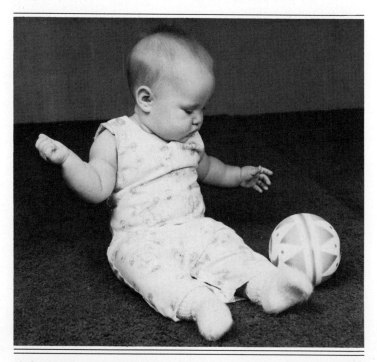

A 9-month-old can sit by herself with a straight back.

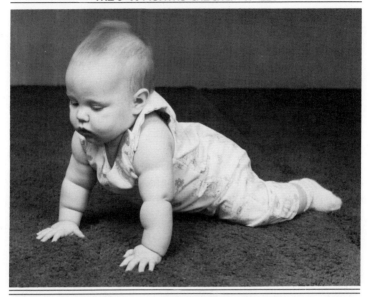

The 9-month-old creeps on hands and knees.
Younger babies crawl—moving forward on
their hands and elbows and dragging their legs.

Now, with her head and trunk under control, it's time for your baby to perfect the control of her extremities. Increasing coordination of legs and feet will lead to standing, climbing, walking (forwards and backwards), and, finally, running. Your baby may already be pulling herself to a standing position (90 percent of babies do so by age 10 months), and if so, she probably holds on to something until she gets tired, then lets herself down, bottom first, with a thump. She may cruise, the term used for walking sideways while holding on to furniture, and she probably walks happily holding on to your hands. A few babies even walk alone at age 9 or 10 months.

Better control of her arms and hands have resulted in increasingly sophisticated movements. Fingers, which once opened and shut together as a mittenlike unit, now work individually. Especially the index finger. This finger has become an inquisitive probe. The eyes of her teddy bear, a green pea on her plate, a new toy, all are approached with the index finger, testing, poking, learning. Learning through handling and mouthing objects continues throughout the first year of life. Primarily everything still goes straight to the mouth, but gradually there will be more manual investigation, more handling of toys and objects, more turning and rotating an object in order to learn more about it.

The index finger, in combination with her thumb, opens up a new world for your 9- to 10-month-old. Before, she could only look at a Cheerio or a piece of puffed rice. Now she can pick it up and get it to her mouth (using her

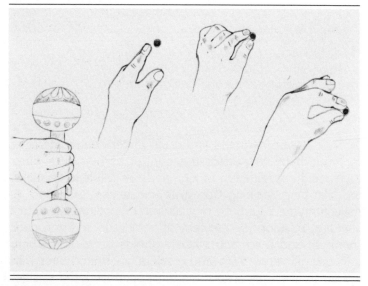

Grasp development (left to right): At age 2 months babies have a mitten grasp, with thumb opposing four fingers. At 9 months the index finger becomes a probe to explore things. At about the same time the pincer grasp develops, allowing the child to pick up a small object between thumb and forefinger while the forearm rests on a flat surface. The fine pincer grasp (right) requires no support from the forearm and develops at about one year.

thumb and forefinger and resting her arm on a flat surface). In a short time, the thumb–finger combination will become a refined pincer grasp (without the need to support her forearm) and there will be no limit to the objects she can pick up to examine or put into her mouth. Unfortunately, that includes buttons, safety pins, and small parts of an older brother or sister's toys. Be sure to keep all such objects out of reach.

Another exciting development that may have occurred by this checkup is that your baby can voluntarily let go of objects. You may recall that until now objects have stayed trapped tightly in her fist until she dropped them by accident. Now, however, she can probably let go on purpose by removing her hand from an object as it rests on a flat surface in front of her. A few precocious 9-month-olds can not only let go of things but can also begin to throw them. More commonly, this is a trait of one-year-olds, and it is discussed in the next chapter.

Personal/Social   If your baby is interested in feeding herself with a spoon, she should be encouraged to do so. There will be plenty of spills and the spoon will be upside down much of the time, but a surprising amount of food will find its way to her mouth if you choose the right kind of food for her to practice with—applesauce, mashed banana, cereal—things that will stick to the spoon. As with other skills, feeding herself is something at which she will quickly become more expert. Most food at this age, of course, is eaten with the fingers.

By 10 months your baby should be overcoming her shyness with strangers. For some parents it has been a very long haul, particularly for those whose babies entered their stranger-anxious period early, at about 5 months of age. Your baby's social accomplishments include playing peek-a-boo and pat-a-cake, and she has probably begun to wave bye-bye as well. Note that she can only play games that allow her to see herself performing the task. With pat-a-cake she can see her own hands. "So big," which requires that she stretch her hands and arms out of sight, won't be accomplished until later.

Language/Communication   Your 9-month-old says "Dada" and "Mama," but she won't really begin to know what that means until she is 10 months old at the earliest. By 10 months she may also have a "word"—one that she made up—that she uses consistently for a single object or food item. Even though her skill with language is yet to come, she is beginning to have a basic understanding of words. She responds to her own name, and she has begun to understand the concept of *no-no,* probably more from the change in tone of your voice than from the actual words.

NUTRITION

This checkup marks the beginning of a change in your baby's physique. Until now she has been building fat, but from now on she'll be building muscle and thinning out a bit. The balance between milk and food changes now, too. Milk is still important, of course, but food is equally important. Your baby should begin to eat three well-balanced meals a day with less milk at each meal and in between meals. In order to establish three meals a day, a limit must be placed on milk. Your doctor may recommend reducing your baby's intake to 16 or 24 ounces a day, depending on how far along she is with her solid foods. Both breast- and bottle-fed babies may be offered milk in a cup along with their meals at this age. This is an important time to introduce the cup if you haven't already done so. At age 9 months the breast-fed baby can be weaned directly to a cup. Commercially prepared or evaporated milk formulas are usually recommended rather than whole cow's milk, which should be withheld for the first year of life.

No matter how well balanced your baby's three daily meals are, she will need between-meal feedings. These snacks may include toast, dry cereal, cheese, or fruit, as well as milk or juice from a cup. Lumpy foods, first introduced at age 6 months, should continue. Some suitable foods are mashed potatoes, cooked carrots, peas, and other vegetables, and small pieces of meat such as liverwurst, ground hamburger, frankfurters, or sausages. Little or no salt should be added in the preparation of foods served to your baby.

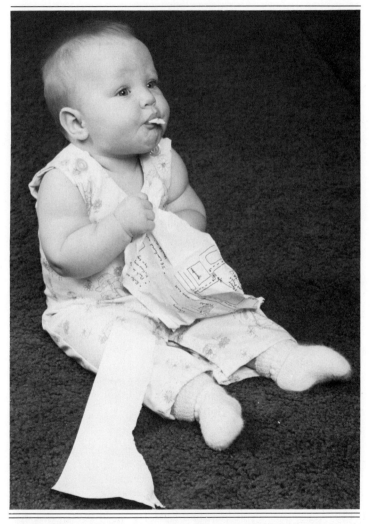

Good nutrition isn't all meat and potatoes.
Sometimes a letter from Grandma tastes good.

When you're counting calories and considering protein for your baby, remember that the word *meat* on the label doesn't tell you how much meat is actually in the jar. Commercial high-meat junior dinners, for example, have *less than half* the protein contained in pure strained meats or junior meats. Commercially prepared vegetable and meat combinations contain *less than one-fifth* as much protein as pure meat. When in doubt, read labels carefully. Although the names are similar, Gerber's Beef with Vegetables is a *high-meat dinner* (one-half the protein of pure meat), whereas Vegetables and Beef is a *vegetable–meat combination* (less than one-fifth the protein of pure meat).

The following chart illustrates the calorie and protein differences among various Gerber products. Note that the vegetable–meat combinations are lower in calories as well as in protein. Keep in mind that the manufacturer isn't trying to trick you, but that you are expected to read the labels on the products you buy. Whatever brand of baby food you choose, there is usually fairly complete information on the labels.

AVERAGE NUTRIENT VALUES PER 100 GRAMS (7 TABLESPOONS)

		Calories	Protein
Junior meats	Beef	98	14.7 g*
	Chicken	137	14.8 g
	Ham	115	15.1 g
Junior high-meat dinners	Beef with Vegetables	98	6.4 g
	Chicken with Vegetables	103	6.8 g
	Ham with Vegetables	82	7.0 g
Junior vegetables and meats	Vegetables & Beef	66	2.8 g
	Vegetables & Chicken	51	2.0 g
	Vegetables & Ham	59	2.3 g

*g = gram

Adapted from Nutrient Values, Gerber Baby Foods, Fremont, Michigan, 1981.

Certain foods should continue to be withheld from your baby. Egg whites and tunafish are allergenic in the first year. There is danger of aspirating (breathing in and choking on) nuts, popcorn, raisins, raw carrots, raw celery, and raw apples. There is danger of choking on marshmallows, taffy, and other sticky foods. Peanut butter by the spoonful is also dangerous. Honey has been implicated in infant botulism in babies less than one year old. Cookies, cakes, and most desserts, whether strained or junior, commercial or prepared at home, are rich in calories and carbohydrates and should be given sparingly to babies and young children.

Some foods are withheld at the discretion of your baby's doctor. A baby who has so far shown no intolerance or allergy to any food may be allowed to have scrambled eggs, for example. Orange juice could be introduced at any time after 6 months, diluted with water at first. Your doctor's prejudice against aspiration foods (those that are inhaled and choked on) may have a lot to do with his personal experience with them. Some doctors don't give a second thought, for instance, to whether or not there are chopped nuts in cookies. One doctor we know, however, had the frightening experience of a child's choking on a nut in the waiting room. Needless to say, his is a no-nonsense, no-nut policy. Aspiration foods can be fatal. Some doctors may ban feeding them to children until they are 3 to 5 years old.

PARENT CONCERNS

(These are only some of the concerns parents have at this checkup. Be sure you have yours written down to discuss with the doctor.)

Bowel Movements   Some of the lumps in baby's food aren't fully digested and are passed in the bowel movements. This is normal.

Discipline   Your baby is too young to be disciplined. She is not being deliberately naughty when she disregards your wishes (not yet, anyway), but is only exploring, at an increasing rate, the world and it boundaries. Try to keep your expectations realistic. The no-no you may have attached to certain objects and activities is quickly forgotten by a 9-month-old. Try to have as few no-no's as possible. That way, there will be limits, but the whole world won't look like a no-no to your child.

Shoes   Shoes are not much use to a 9-month-old, even to those few who are already beginning to walk alone. Babies feel much more secure when their toes are free to grip the floor, and traditional, high-top, hard-soled shoes aren't constructed for that kind of freedom. A better choice would be rubber-soled sneakers. These are soft, flexible, lightweight, and nonslip. Even babies seem to appreciate their status value as the shoe of choice for young people. As for siblings' shoes—a pair of sneakers or shoes outgrown by an older brother or sister—some doctors think it won't hurt to let your baby wear them if they fit well and aren't too worn.

Toilet Training   It is true that your baby sits up well by herself, is more observant of her surroundings, and is somewhat more aware of your wishes than when she was an infant. It may even be true that she has bowel movements reasonably regularly and that she urinates within a predicatable time after drinking milk or juice. Does all this add up to readiness for toilet training? No. It's much too soon. You would only be training yourself to play catch at the appropriate times. As for baby, she is months away from being able to make the mental and physical connections necessary for toilet training.

REMINDERS

Safety Topics   Home accidents—poisons, falls, burns, and small objects in the mouth. See Chapter 3.

Appetite   Look for a gradual drop in your baby's appetite between now and the next checkup. This is normal. It happens because of a slowing in the growth process that is beginning to occur now. Your baby has to slow down. She couldn't possibly continue to grow at the rate she's been going since birth or she would soon be as big as Godzilla.

Toys   Bath toys, plastic beach balls, books with stiff pages, old magazines.

CALLING THE DOCTOR

With your baby's increasing physical achievement and capacity for getting into mischief, it's time to think not only of when to call the doctor but also of when it might be even better to call upon other emergency resources in your community.

When an injury or illness is severe, your child should be taken directly to a hospital emergency room. Discuss with your doctor the hospital emergency room he would like you to use and the conditions under which he would like you to use it. The emergency room he recommends will no doubt be one with complete medical and surgical services, fully staffed on a 24-hour basis. It may be located at a children's hospital. In any case, the time to discuss it is now, before you need it. Injuries and symptoms that may require immediate attention in an emergency room rather than in the doctor's office include

- Bleeding that can't be stopped
- Near-drowning
- Falls that result in unconsciousness or cause bleeding from the ears, nose, or mouth
- Seizures, severe breathing difficulties, or baby difficult to arouse
- High (103–104°) fever with baby also appearing to be quite sick
- Accidental poisoning

When poison is accidentally swallowed by a family member, your first telephone call should be to the poison information or control center if there is one in your community. If not, call the doctor or a hospital emergency room. Keep by your telephone the telephone numbers of your doctor, poison-control center, and ambulance service. Remember to take the poison container to the telephone with you so that you can read its contents to the person who answers the phone. Different kinds of poisons require different kinds of first aid.

NEXT CHECKUP

Your baby's next checkup will be in three months, when she is a year old. Watch for the following physical developments between now and then. (Details are in the next chapter.)

- Walks or cruises
- Creeps upstairs (Watch out for this one! Falls are a danger.)
- Climbs into small chair to sit
- Throws things

10
THE ONE-YEAR
CHECKUP

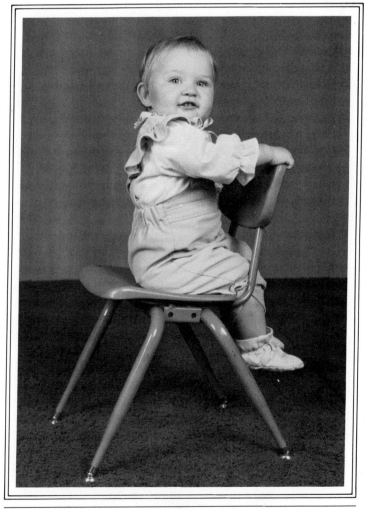

✓ CHECKLIST

ONE-YEAR CHECKUP

Date _____

Procedures

_____ Weigh and measure   Weight _____
                                           Percentile _____
                                              Height _____
                                          Percentile _____
                            Head circumference _____

_____ Discuss height and weight gains on
        growth charts with parents

_____ Cover test (for crossed eyes)
        if not done previously

_____ Tuberculosis test

_____ Hematocrit (Hct)/Hemoglobin (Hgb)
        if not done previously

_____ Discuss nutrition

_____ Ask about parent concerns

_____ Counsel on safety

PHYSICAL EXAMINATION*

Special attention to:

_____ Hearing

_____ Vision

_____ Developmental milestones
        (walks or cruises, stands alone)

_____ Feet and legs in standing position

_____ Spine, standing and sitting

_____ Mouth for teeth

*The complete physical examination is described and illustrated in Chapter 4.

At age one your baby reaches a landmark. She is no longer an infant, but a child. The routine for weighing and measuring her doesn't change, despite her new grownup status, however. She is still usually weighed on the "baby" scales, for some toddlers find the wobbly base on the adult scales frightening to stand on. Also, her height is still measured while she is lying on her back. The recumbent position will continue at least until she is age 2.

A more accurate measurement is possible when the child is lying down. When people stand, including little people, there is compression of the vertebrae in the spinal column of the back that causes them to shrink down a bit. That means we are all literally taller lying down than we are standing up. Further, children under the age of 2 years don't stand up straight. They have a special kind of posture, called lordosis, that doesn't make for accurate measurements when standing. They have pronounced swayed backs and pot bellies, both of which are normal and disappear sometime after age 2. In the meantime, a measurement lying down is a truer measure.

There is an expected weight and height gain for one-year-olds. The "average" baby triples her birthweight at this age and increases her birth height by 50 percent. So if your baby weighed eight pounds at birth and was 20 inches long, she will now weigh *roughly* 24 pounds and be 30 inches tall. The average head circumference at one year is 47 centimeters, which is 18½ inches. All of this is rule of thumb, of course, not exact science because, as everybody knows, there's no such thing as an average baby.

A skin test for tuberculosis is recommended at age one year. Your child may already have had this test if you live in a geographic area where the incidence of TB is greater than one percent or if your child was known to be exposed to the disease. It is possible that other tests will be done at this checkup as well. During the first year of life several tests are performed at the doctor's discretion, some of which your child may not yet have had. These include the cover test and the hematocrit or hemoglobin tests. The cover (and uncover) test is an eye test to help identify babies with crossed or lazy eyes. The hematocrit and hemoglobin are blood tests that determine the percentage of red blood cells in order to identify iron deficiency anemia. All these tests are described more fully in earlier chapters.

Babies at high risk for lead poisoning are also tested at about this age. This includes youngsters who live in old housing units where the flaking and chipping from many layers of lead-based paints can be a serious health risk. Lead poisoning is discussed in Chapter 3.

Until recently, all babies were innoculated against smallpox at the one-year checkup. This is no longer either recommended or performed, however, because the disease has virtually been eliminated from the planet, a fact officially observed by the World Health Organization (WHO) in 1979. Should smallpox ever become a problem again, of course, routine innoculations would immediately be reinstated.

THE PHYSICAL EXAMINATION

Your baby will probably be checked over thoroughly by means of a physical examination such as the one described in Chapter 4. The least disturbing maneuvers are often done first, the ones that don't require instruments. Usually the examiner accommodates himself to the baby's mood. Much can be accomplished by allowing an anxious tot to remain in her mother's lap. No doctor wants to get into a wrestling match with a frightened or angry child, so most would rather skip a maneuver than force it on a truly uncooperative patient, especially if that maneuver has not yielded any abnormal findings in the past. The doctor will simply make note of his failure and try again next time.

Your child's mouth will be checked for teeth. It is normal for a one-year-old to have as many as six or eight teeth or as few as two.

The doctor probably looks into your baby's nose with the otoscope routinely at each well baby checkup. Until now he's been looking primarily for obstructions and congestion. As of this checkup, though, he's also on the lookout for foreign bodies. Your child, remember, now has a neat pincer grasp. That means she is skilled at picking up really small objects between her thumb and forefinger . . . and stuffing them up her nose. Foreign bodies recovered from babies' noses include raisins, buttons, uninflated balloons,

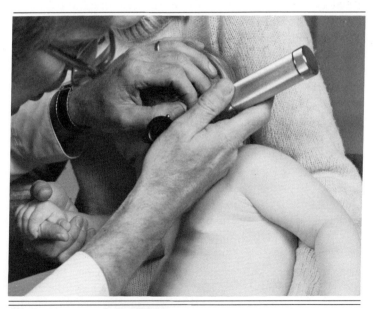

If a child is anxious, much of the physical examination can be performed with her in her mother's lap.

green beans, and erasers, just to name a few. These objects are sometimes, but not usually, discovered at routine checkups. More often, the parents take the child to the doctor either because they have seen her put the object in her nose or because the resulting bad odor and foul discharge from her nose.

The baby's eyes are checked with both the ophthalmoscope and penlight for the red reflex and for pupillary response to light, both described in Chapter 4. The doctor may also ask if your baby seems to see well and if she seems to pay attention to what she sees. He must depend on your observations because the child isn't old enough yet to take a vision test. For older children there are Snellen charts, which have E's in various sizes and positions. The child demonstrates her vision by pointing her finger in the direction the E is going. There are variations on this test designed for young children, but a one-year-old isn't old enough for these tests. Meanwhile, the doctor must depend on you to report how well you think your child sees.

To repeat from previous chapters—warning signs of poor vision in a child are that she always brings objects very close to her face when looking at them. Other signs are closing or covering one eye or constantly leaning forward in an effort to see better. She may also wrinkle her face, so intense is her straining to see.

When the doctor examines the child's ear with an otoscope, he will be on the lookout now for foreign objects that she may have stuck there—the same ones that get put into the nose. Also of concern is the occasional insect that finds its way into the ear canal. The doctor may ask if the child seems to hear, and more important, if she seems to understand what she hears.

A child with impaired hearing may be able to hear loud sounds but be unable to hear words spoken in a normal tone of voice. Such a child might also turn her head to a preferred side when listening. Clues to your child's being able to hear well are whether or not she appears to be listening to you when you speak and whether she responds to her name or to a whispered command like "Give me the ball" when her back is turned to you. Another clue to her hearing is the distinctness of her developing speech. Children who don't hear well tend to drop the endings of words because they don't hear them. Even children with normal hearing mispronounce words, of course, sometimes because of parental reinforcement. If, for example, your child's first attempt at the word breakfast comes out *bahkoos,* and you think it's cute and invite her to *bahkoos* each morning, *bahkoos* it will be for quite a long time. Generally, it isn't a good idea to speak or encourage too much baby talk. All of it will eventually have to be corrected and relearned by the child, and it really isn't helpful to the development of normal speech.

The doctor will probably ask about your child's vocabulary. The range of normal for a one-year-old includes everything from just *Dada* to four or five other words with meaning. Babies are a lot like tape recorders. Whatever you say repeatedly to them tends to be "played back" by the child. So do words that you reinforce. If you get all excited when she says *"Dada,"* she will certainly say it more frequently. Unfortunately, babies are indiscriminate about the words they pick up and play back. Their speech reflects their social contacts, and when those include one or two worldy-wise siblings, the results can be startling. One cherubic 2-year-old girl with two older brothers, seated at brunch one morning with her parents and visiting grandparents, was heard to inquire sweetly, "Dammit, where is my toast?"

MILESTONES IN DEVELOPMENT ± *

Motor/Physical
- Stands alone briefly
- Cruises, may walk alone or with one hand held
- Creeps upstairs
- Climbs onto furniture

*The plus-or-minus sign indicates that your child may very well reach developmental milestones earlier or later than what is indicated here as "average." There is a wide range of normal in child development.

- Has neat pincer grasp
- Lets go of objects voluntarily

Personal/Social
- Drinks from cup (spills)
- Throws a ball
- Points, indicates wants without crying
- Drools less
- Mouths objects less

Language/Communication
- Says "Dada, Mama" with meaning
- Says two or three other words and appears to understand meaning of several more
- Understands meaning of simple phrases

The doctor will either check or ask about some, not all, of the above milestones during the one-year checkup. Some are listed for your own interest because your knowledge of development and your expectations for your child have much to do with her progress. Working with your child with a positive attitude will help her to develop her full potential.

Motor/Physical   When the doctor examines your toddler for motor development at this checkup, he is looking particularly for her ability to stand alone and/or walk. One way or another, the one-year-old walks. You may remember that the progress of human development is from head to foot (cephalocaudal). With her head, body, and hands in pretty good control, your baby is now concentrating on her legs, feet, and walking skills. She may cruise (walk holding on to furniture), walk holding one of your hands, or walk alone. The range of normal for walking alone is from 9 months to 16 months with some overflow on either end. That is, the occasional baby will walk even earlier than 9 months or later than 16 months. The doctor will probably have the child walk toward you during the examination so that he can observe her gait, the way she walks.

Watching her walk is the best way for the doctor to discover abnormal posture of her legs. He is also checking for limping, weakness, stiffness of joints, or limited range of

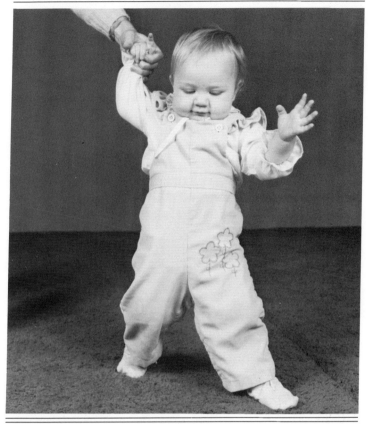

One way or another, the one-year-old walks—either alone, with one hand held, or holding onto furniture (cruising).

motion that would suggest a problem. He wants to be sure, too, that she walks with her feet flat on the floor. She should no longer walk on her toes.

Sometimes toddlers develop a painful and very tender elbow. Called nursemaid's elbow, it comes from the child's having been pulled to a standing position by one arm or lifted up a step or over a curb. Children should be lifted instead with equal weight under both arms to avoid this kind of injury. The doctor can correct the injury by means of a simple maneuver that can be done in the office, but it is better avoided.

You may have noticed that your child can pivot her body now. When she's standing or sitting, she can turn to look over her shoulder or reach for an object behind her. Pivoting, or rotation, is the most sophisticated movement in human motor development. As such, it's one of the final movements to be mastered in each body skill area. Walking, for example, is actually the ultimate in rotational movement, a series of complex rotating movements involving the hips, legs, and torso.

Likewise, chewing is the ultimate in rotational jaw movement. When you chew, your jaws move not only up and down, but they also rotate. Your baby's jaws are also beginning to rotate when she chews. Until now, though, she

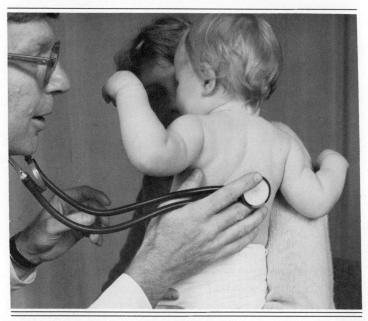

The one-year-old can pivot her body,
a sign of normal physical development.

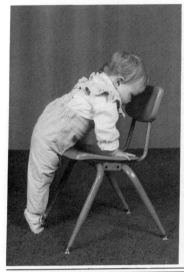 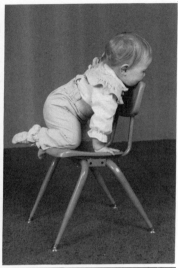

The fact that one-year-olds love to climb is not hard to understand when you consider how long they've been looking at the world from shin level.

chewed with only up-and-down motion. Because of this developing sophistication of jaw movement, it will be easier for her to chew tougher substances like meat, and they won't have to be chopped quite so fine.

Another oral development is that a one-year-old can move her tongue laterally to the corner of her mouth to lick off a piece of food. Previously she could only move her tongue in and out of her mouth in a straight line.

Your year-old not only walks, but she probably also climbs. Getting a leg up, reaching toward the towering grownup world, seems to be very much on the minds of most one-year-olds. When they're not climbing stairs on all fours, they're climbing into adult chairs and onto tables and sofas. This is not difficult to understand, really, when you consider how long a time your baby has spent looking at the world from shin level. Stairs are fascinating and great fun as long as you are there to supervise. Baby can creep up the stairs easily, but getting down is not so easy. The safety gates on your stairs at home should remain in place for a while longer.

The one-year-old has mastered basic hand and finger movements. She now has what is called a neat pincer grasp. That means she can pick up a small object from above the object with her thumb and index finger, zooming down on it with the precision of a helicopter. Previously she

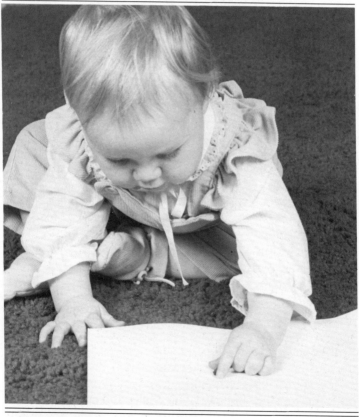

Having mastered basic hand and finger movements, the one-year-old can pick up a small object between thumb and index finger. This is called the pincer grasp.

had to rest her forearm on a flat surface in order to use the thumb–finger combination.

When you read to your child now, she probably tries to help turn the pages and seems to enjoy herself thoroughly. Reading to her and allowing her to have books of her own are very important. She enjoys the pictures in magazines as well and may spend quite long periods playing with them quietly and turning the pages. She'll also rip them up, so be sure to give her old ones and remember that some messy play is not only okay but really essential to her growth and development.

One of the most exciting things that is happening to your child physically is that she can now voluntarily let go of, drop, and even throw objects. She's probably been tossing toys out of her crib and playpen and off the tray of her high chair. This deceptively simple (and sometimes annoying) act is really the final accomplishment in an evolution of personal achievement for your child. Called casting, it may develop as early as 8 months, reaching its height at 12 to 15 months.

Human development is an orderly, predictable process, and all babies go through it one step at a time. The evolution in this case was reach ⟶ grasp ⟶ release, which sounds a lot more complicated than it really is.

Gaining control of her extremities is an important part of your child's motor development. Third in the development process, it follows head and body/trunk control. At age 4 months she developed good head control and, almost simultaneously, enough control of her body to sit upright with some support. She was not so clever with her hands yet, though, and when an object excited her interest she could only swipe at it, usually missing it by a country mile.

Soon, at age 6 months, she could reach accurately for an object and grasp it in her hand. But having grasped it, she still didn't know how to let go. (Remember how you stuck your finger in her fist when she was a newborn and she seemed to hang on forever? That was because she couldn't let go.) Even at 9 months, although she knew how to remove her hand from an object resting on a flat surface, she probably didn't know how to drop it deliberately.

Now at last she knows how. And how! She's gone through the predictable stages of reach——→grasp——→ release. She's tossing toys, dishes, spoons, and anything else she can get her hands on, and you may be impatient with having to pick them up. It might help to look at her throwing things as a celebration of an important motor accomplishment rather than as a pain in the neck. Besides, she'll stop behaving like a major-league baseball pitcher at about 15 months of age, if not sooner. That, too, is part of the orderly process of development.

Personal/Social By age one year, about half of all babies can drink from a cup, either with assistance or by

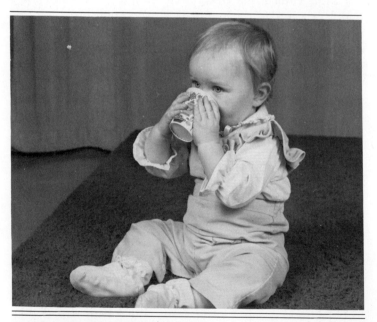

By age one year, about half of all babies can drink from a cup, either by themselves or with some assistance.

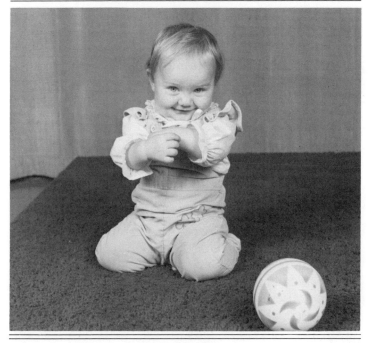

*The one-year-old can throw
a ball to another person.*

themselves. Most of their fluids—milk, juice, or water—
should be taken by a cup at this age, saving bottle or
breast-feedings for early waking and bedtime feedings.
There is still some spilling when the baby drinks from a cup,
but on the whole it is becoming a fairly neat process. Your
baby is also becoming a better communicator. She can
point to something and indicate she wants it without whin-
ing or crying.

She can also throw a ball. Although this requires
motor skill, it also rates as a social development because it
requires understanding and cooperating with another person. She cooperates when being dressed as well, moving
her arms and body to help out.

You will notice that your baby is drooling less and that she is also mouthing objects much less than she used to. This has a lot to do with her newly developed skill with hands and fingers. Both are much more dexterous at exploring objects than they were before, so it has become more interesting for her to handle an object—twist it, turn it, shake it, drop it, pick it back up, turn it upside down—than it is to mouth it.

Language/Communication   Your baby probably uses *Dada* and *Mama* meaningfully, along with two or three other words. Among the most popular ones are *up, bye-bye, all gone, more, there,* and *that.* It is interesting to note that these are all words that can be used universally to describe any object. As such, they are extremely useful to a baby. She can say "all gone" to refer to Daddy, a dog, a butterfly, or the food on her plate. In addition to being able to say two or three words, a one-year-old usually knows the meaning of several more. She also understands the meaning of simple phrases like "Where is your shoe?" or "Don't touch." She may also have a few "words" of her own invention that she uses regularly.

NUTRITION

With your child's first birthday comes a landmark in nutrition. The transitional period between infant and adult eating patterns is now officially over, and it's time for her to eat like a grownup—almost. Some precautions persist. It is still wise to be stingy with sugar and salt to help your child avoid developing tastes for either—sugar because it is a decayer of teeth and producer of fat and fat cells, and salt because it has been implicated in high blood pressure, stroke, and heart disease. It is also wise to continue to withhold aspiration foods, foods that may be inhaled and choked on—raisins, popcorn, all kinds of nuts, raw carrots, celery, and apples.

Peanut butter eaten by the spoonful may also be extremely hazardous. A wad of peanut butter stuck in the trachea (windpipe) behaves like glue. It is simply not possible to dislodge it by any conventional emergency method. Peanut butter spread *thinly* on bread or a cracker poses no such hazard, provided it is the smooth, not the chunky, variety.

The ban on honey can now be lifted. Since it has been implicated in cases of botulism poisoning in infants less than one year of age, it is not recommended sooner. Highly allergenic in younger babies, eggs too can be introduced now if the doctor recommends them. He may already have introduced egg yolk into your baby's diet, for it is egg whites that usually cause allergies. Some doctors suggest restricting the number of eggs per week to three or four because of their high cholesterol level, although the cholesterol controversy has still not been settled by medical researchers.

Your child's daily menu need be limited only by your imagination. Anything cut into bite-size pieces will probably be well received—bread, luncheon meat, cheese, fruit—anything that can be picked up and eaten with the hands. Give your child some practice with a spoon, too, but don't expect miracles. A one-year-old reflexively turns the spoon upside down just as it reaches her mouth. She can't help it; it just happens. That's why it's so important that you choose foods for spooning that will stick to the spoon—cereal, thick soup, mashed potatoes mixed with vegetables, etc.

Each day the baby's meals should include servings of something from each of the four basic food groups—three or more servings of milk and milk products (cheese, cottage cheese, yogurt), four servings of grains (cereal, bread, crackers), four servings of fruits and vegetables, and two or more servings of meat. There's no mystery to this, and it's quite easy to achieve. A typical day's menu might look something like this.

Breakfast   Juice, cereal, and milk

Lunch   Quarter slice bread, spread thinly with peanut butter and cut into small pieces, cooked carrot sticks, milk

Snacks   Choose one: cheese strips, oven-dried toast, small pieces of vegetable; fruit juice

Dinner   Ground meat, mashed potatoes, cooked vegetables, fruit, and milk

This easy menu provides three servings from the milk group, three from the grain group, four from the fruit/ vegetable group, and two from the meat group. (High in protein, peanut butter counts in the meat group.)

The goal at mealtimes is to serve a variety of foods that are suited to the baby's chewing capabilities. Because her chewing is not quite mature yet (rotation of the jaw is just now developing), meat still has to be chopped fairly finely in order for her to be able to handle it. The secret to introducing new foods is to introduce them at a time when the baby is very hungry and to give them small amounts, accompanied by a food she likes.

Choose snack foods that are low in sugar and fat so they don't spoil the baby's appetite for her next scheduled meal. Appropriate are fruit juices or small pieces of fruit, small pieces of raw vegetables (not carrots, celery, or apples), small pieces of cheese with cracker, or a small portion of bread or toast.

What to feed the baby is relatively easy. Letting her decide for herself how much she wants to eat may not be quite as easy. It's very hard for parents to resist being members of the clean-plate club, but try you must. Your child knows when she's had enough, just as she did when she was an infant. And just as you respected that then, you must continue to respect it now. Remember that her enormous growth spurt is slowing markedly and that she doesn't require the constant feeding that she once did. A dropoff in appetite at age one year is normal and to be expected. If you turn to the growth charts at the back of the book, you will see that the steep rise in rate of growth and weight begins to fall off at about age 9 months.

Try not to overwhelm your baby with the size of the portions on her plate. Most important, remember that no normal, healthy baby has ever starved to death. Most babies can be depended upon to eat when they are hungry. If, however, you are truly concerned that your baby eats "less than she should," mention it to the doctor. Parents are sometimes asked to keep food records in order to document or disprove a true feeding problem.

Portions that might be considered average-sized for a one-year-old include

Cereal	¼ cup
Potato Macaroni Spaghetti	¼ cup
Vegetables	1–2 tablespoons
Fruits	¼ cup
Eggs	1
Meats Fish without bones Cheese	¼ to 1 ounce

A rule of thumb is that the child will be eating 7 to 10 tablespoons of various solids at each of the three meals plus smaller servings of low-sugar snacks.

Vitamins The doctor may take your baby off supplemental vitamins now, although some doctors recommend that they be continued for a while longer. There is support for both viewpoints. The case for continuing vitamins is that the child will be switching now from breast milk or formula to a controlled amount of regular cow's milk, which contains fewer vitamins than formula does. The argument against continuing vitamins is that a child who is fed three well-balanced meals a day is getting all the vitamins she needs. Vitamins are not harmful in normal doses, but most youngsters who eat citrus fruits, don't live in the Arctic, and aren't starved for long periods of time do not need vitamins after age one year.

Milk If your baby is breast-fed, one or both of you may decide to stop at any time now. At this age, the baby should be weaned directly to a cup, and milk intake should be limited to 16 ounces (half a quart) a day. Children who routinely drink more than that may be offered water or juice to drink as a substitute. Although skim or whole milk is acceptable at this age in that amount, your doctor may suggest formula instead if your child has shown allergies or food intolerance in the past.

If your baby is bottle-fed, it's time to encourage most of the 16-ounce limit to be taken from a cup. As with breast-fed babies, the doctor may suggest a switch to whole cow's milk now. One-year-olds need assistance with their drinking from a cup. They don't become really skilled at it until about 17 months of age. Meanwhile, cups with lids and weighted bottoms are useful.

One last thing about food and one-year-olds is that this age group is messy when they eat, which sometimes creates a conflict with parents, who wish their children could be neater. Your one-year-old will certainly be neater in time, but meanwhile it is very important that she feeds herself—messy or not—because it helps her develop self-reliance.

PARENT CONCERNS

(These are only some of the concerns parents have at this checkup. Be sure you have yours written down to discuss with the doctor.)

Appetite   There is a natural dropoff in the rate of growth. Consider that your baby has tripled her birthweight in one year. During the coming year, however, she is expected to gain only five or six pounds. Consider, too, that she has increased her height at birth about 10 inches this past year. But she will grow only about 5 inches in the coming year. Her brain growth will slow, too, as indicated by the increase in the circumference of her head. While it increased more than 4 inches in the first year, this coming year it will increase only about ¾ of an inch (2 cm).

Discipline   You need to set limits for your child. Know about substitution, the fine art of distracting a baby from an undesirable activity or object by substituting an acceptable one. But be fair. If there's a porcelain figurine in your house that continually attracts the baby's attention, move it beyond her reach permanently rather than trying to enforce a no-no concerning it. Think of it from the baby's point of view. She sees the figurine (or crystal vase, or

Daddy's reading glasses, or whatever) and goes for it. Much to her delight, she can make a whole roomful of protesting grownups mobilize to rescue the object. That's so much fun that she wants to repeat the experience. So don't make a big deal of the rescue; just take the object away from her, give her a toy in its place, and put the object permanently out of her reach. Remember that it is vital to your child's development that she explore her surroundings and that everything in them should not be a no-no.

Shoes   Traditional high-top, hard-soled shoes are appropriate now if your doctor recommends them. The soles are slippery at first, so it's a good idea to rough them up by hand on a course surface such as a sidewalk or patio. You can also apply a piece of cloth adhesive tape to the soles to add traction. High tops are *not* healthier for your child's feet than other kinds of shoes. They offer only one advantage over softer shoes like sneakers. They are harder for the child to remove by herself. Taking off shoes is a favorite toddler activity that parents sometimes lose patience with.

A properly fitted shoe should have a thumb's-width growing room between the child's toe and the end of the shoe. *But it should be the width of the child's thumb, not the salesperson's.* As for the width of the shoe, you should be able to pinch a little bit of it, between your fingers to ensure it isn't too narrow.

Toilet Training   Your doctor will probably tell you to wait until the child is at least 18 months old before attempting to toilet-train her.

REMINDERS

Safety Topics   Accidents that come with greater mobility. See Chapter 3 for details.

Communication   Talk to your baby. Read to her often. Show her pictures and name objects for her continually. This is the way she develops her language skills.

Tooth Care   If your child has the minimum number of teeth (two), you may continue to care for them with the wiping method described in Chapter 9. If she has as many as eight teeth, however, you may choose to begin caring for them with a toothbrush. Vistron-Pro makes Pro Guard, an orange-flavored toothbrush with soft bristles suitable for children from ages one to four years, and there are other toothbrushes your dentist can recommend as well. Hints on how to brush your child's teeth are included in Chapter 12.

Toys   Toys that involve putting one piece in another. Pull toys if baby walks. Balls.

NEXT CHECKUP

You will be asked to bring your child to the office at age 15 months for immunization against measles, mumps, and rubella (German measles) and possibly for a checkup as well. Whether or not a checkup is included with the shot will depend on the schedule maintained by the office.

By age 15 months your youngster will be walking very well alone and may even be running. Be on guard for this new mobility and the dangers that go along with it.

Watch for these additional landmarks in development. (Details are in the next chapter.)

• Walks upstairs, one hand held
• Stoops to pick up toy
• Likes to take off shoes
• Points to one or more body parts

RESOURCES

Tel Med,   free tape-recorded health information by telephone, has many titles of interest to parents of children between the ages of 1 and 2 years. See the "Resources" section at the end of Chapter 5 for further details.

Ross Laboratories   booklets available to parents in the offices of pediatricians include *The Single-Parent Family, Your Baby Becomes a Toddler, Your Child's Appetite,* and—for the older child (15 months to 2 years)— *Developing Toilet Habits, Your Children and Discipline, When Your Child Is Contrary, When Your Child Is Unruly,* and *Your Child's Fears.*

11
THE 15-MONTHS
CHECKUP

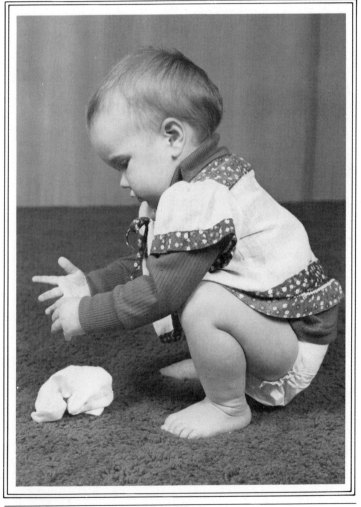

✓ CHECKLIST

15-MONTHS CHECKUP

Date _____

Procedures

_____ Weigh and Measure

Weight _____

Percentile _____

Height _____

Percentile _____

Head circumference _____

_____ Discuss weight and height gains on growth charts with parents

_____ MMR/Immunization against measles, mumps, and rubella (German measles)

_____ Cover test (for crossed eyes) if not done previously

_____ Hematocrit (Hct)/Hemoglobin (Hgb) if not done previously

_____ Discuss nutrition

_____ Ask about parent concerns

_____ Counsel on safety

PHYSICAL EXAMINATION*

Special attention to:

_____ Hearing

_____ Vision

_____ Gait

_____ Spine, standing and sitting

_____ Mouth for teeth

_____ Developmental milestones (walks, runs)

*The complete physical examination is described and illustrated in Chapter 4.

With their brand-new physical abilities and their desire to do so much so vigorously, 15-month-olds are known to the doctors who take care of them as the dart-dash-or-fling bunch. Most of them don't hold still for long, forcing the examiner to accommodate himself to whatever position the youngster happens to be in at the moment. This is usually no handicap for the clever examiner, who can get much of the information he needs by observing the child, by performing maneuvers quickly and skillfully, and by getting help from the parents for procedures that require the patient to be on the examining table or holding still. The doctor also depends on parents to report a certain amount of important information, especially in matters of nutrition and motor development.

If you have an active toddler, there's no reason to expect she'll magically quiet down for a physical examination. If she squirms and fidgets or wants to get up and walk around, she's not being naughty; she's just being normal. Nor is it naughty for her to resist some of the examination maneuvers. That, too, is normal.

At about this age, doctors begin to communicate directly with their small patients. The doctor will probably talk to your child in a calm, quiet voice, explaining each step in the examination process to her. He will say, "I am going to look in your ear." He will *not* say, "Is it all right if I look in your ear?" because we all know what the answer to that would be. It's important to keep up communication with a 15-month-old child who is being examined, not only because she understands quite a bit but also because it can help to relieve her anxiety and reduce any conflict with the examiner.

It certainly won't erase her fears completely, but it is only fair to make her an integral part of her own examination, to the limit of her understanding. One takes the time, after all, to explain to her what is going on in picture books, and a physical examination is much more immediate and important to her than that. That's why some doctors give toddlers the tongue depressor to hold after they've examined the mouth, for example. And most talk the child through each procedure as it is performed.

THE PHYSICAL EXAMINATION

Even though it is somewhat catch-as-catch-can, the exam will include most, if not all, of the procedures described in Chapter 4, although counting the femoral pulses in the groin is usually discontinued at this age. The hips may continue to be abducted through age 2, checking for dislocation problems. Examination of the mouth will reveal about nine teeth, although the number of teeth remains highly variable. A check of the head for the anterior fontanel (the soft spot on top) will probably show that it has either grown very small or is closed by now. Closure normally occurs by 18 months, although it can occur any time between 9 and 18 months.

In order to check her gait, the doctor will probably have your youngster walk toward you a short distance while he stands behind her, watching the way she walks. Normally the 15-month-old walks with her legs somewhat wide apart and is a little bit unstable. There should be no toeing-in, limping, or walking on the tips of her toes. Toeing-out should also have disappeared by now.

The final act of the examination will be to immunize your child against measles, mumps, and rubella (German measles) and to answer any questions you have about the innoculation. All three vaccines are customarily given as a single shot into the large muscle of the thigh.

Immunization against measles, mumps, and rubella is

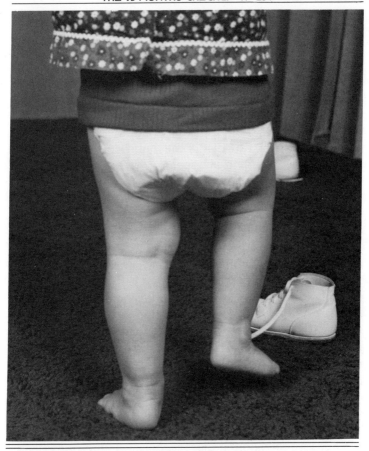

"Walk to Mom" is usually the last item in every physical checkup. This is the way the doctor checks the child's gait, the way she walks.

recommended at age 15 months by the American Academy of Pediatrics. All three are highly contagious viral diseases that affect children primarily. By means of antibodies they received from their mothers, babies have immunity against these illnesses that lasts anywhere from four to six or eight months before it begins to be lost. Babies younger than age 15 months apparently cannot make antibodies as successfully as they do later. That is why inoculation is delayed until age 15 months.

Measles and mumps are both acute childhood illnesses that can also cause serious complications. As for rubella, although it causes only mild illness in the children who contract it, its effect on unborn babies is devastating. When an expectant mother is exposed to the disease in the first three months of her pregnancy, there is danger of miscarriage, stillbirth, or—if the baby survives—multiple birth defects, including blindness, deafness, and heart disease.

Measles, too, can be serious. It always causes high fever of 104–105°F, and during the height of the fever the child is extremely ill. Measles can also cause pneumonia and ear infections. Other complications include deafness, blindness, and encephalitis (inflammation of the brain tissue). Encephalitis is fatal in 10 percent of cases. Mumps not only causes fever and painful swelling of salivary glands in the neck, but it can also cause pancreatitis (inflammation of the pancreas), meningitis (inflammation of the membrane lining of the brain), and permanent deafness.

The Vaccines Measles, mumps, and German measles are all viral diseases, and the vaccines that protect against them are all made from live, although weakened (attenuated), viruses. In this way the body is encouraged to produce antibodies and immunization against disease without actually causing the disease. Measles and mumps vaccines are prepared in cultures of chicken embryo cells; rubella (German measles) vaccine is prepared in cell cultures from birds and mammals, including humans.

Risks and Reactions to the Vaccines Measles, mumps, and rubella vaccines are usually given in combination as a single shot, although they are available singly. Licensed since 1963, measles vaccine has proved to be safe and highly effective based on the results of more than 80 million doses that have been given in the United States and abroad since that time. A single dose is effective 95 percent of the time, providing permanent immunization against the disease. Ten to 20 percent of immunized children may develop a moderate fever of between 101 and 103°F and, less commonly, rash within 5 to 12 days. One person in a million may develop encephalitis as a result of vaccination. Although that is certainly a serious consideration for parents, it should be weighed against the fact that *one in* 1,000 babies develops encephalitis with natural measles. That means your baby's risk of measles-related encephalitis is 1,000 times greater from measles than it is from measles vaccination.

Ideally, measles vaccine should be given either at the same time or after tuberculosis testing is done. Given before TB testing, it can cause a temporary loss of accurate response to the TB test. Although the best age for measles immunization is 15 months, it may be necessary to give it as early as age 6 or 9 months to children who live in areas where the incidence of measles is high. In those cases a second dose should be given after age 15 months.

A single dose of mumps vaccine provides full protection from the disease to 90 percent of those who receive it. Reactions to the vaccination can include fever and swelling of the salivary glands a week or two after the shot, but both are rare. Mumps vaccine should not be given to pregnant women. Although the risk to the unborn baby is not known, virus from the vaccine has been shown to cross the placenta to the fetus.

More than 70 million children have been vaccinated against German measles since rubella vaccine was licensed in 1969. A single dose is effective 90 percent of the time, and there are no serious risks associated with vaccination. About one in seven children develops rash or swollen glands within a week or two of the shot. Occasionally there is temporary joint pain (arthralgia) in about 1 percent of children, with a higher percentage in teenagers. Sometimes moderate fever lymph involvement (lymphadenopathy) occur, and rarely, rash. Rubella vaccine is not given to babies less than a year old because they do not form antibodies well before age one. It should not be given to females of childbearing age who will not be protected from pregnancy for a full three months.

Chicken pox, also called varicella, is another common childhood disease. Although it usually affects children between ages 5 and 9 years, it can be contracted by children of any age, including infants, and by adults as well. Unlike measles, mumps, and rubella, there has been no vaccine developed for chicken pox in the United States

Remember that immunizations are available either free of charge or at reduced cost from your local health department. And don't forget to add this immunization to the permanent records provided at the back of this book.

MILESTONES IN DEVELOPMENT ± *

Motor/Physical
- Walks well, falls little
- Runs stiffly
- Walks upstairs, one hand held
- Stoops to pick up toy
- Throws ball

Personal/Social
- Drinks from cup
- Uses spoon (still spills)
- Likes to take off shoes
- Seeks help from another

Language
- *Mama, Dada* plus three to ten other words
- Points to one or more body parts
- Says "thank you" (although may use a substitute word)

Although almost all babies walk alone by the time they are 15 months old, there are a few cautious holdouts who wait a while longer, and it is perfectly normal for them to do so. If your child isn't walking alone yet, her readiness can be judged by her cruising between pieces of furniture, by her ability to stand alone for a few seconds, and by her ability to

---

*The plus-or-minus sign indicates that your child may very well reach developmental milestones earlier or later than what is indicated here as "average." There is a wide range of normal in child development.

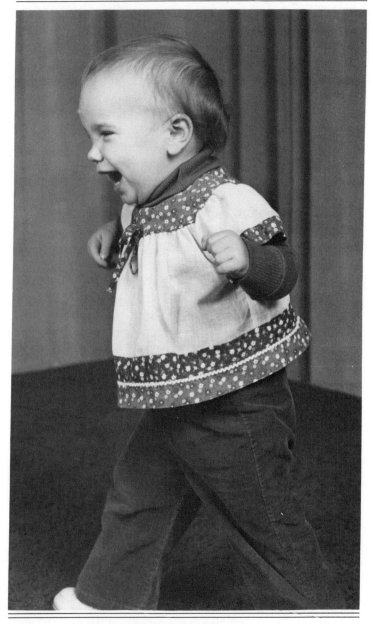

*Fifteen-month-old toddlers walk with their
hands held above waist level for balance.*

walk with one hand held. All of these indicate normal patterns of walking development.

The term *toddler* may come from the very special way that 15-month-old youngsters walk. They toddle along like little wind-up toys, their arms and hands held waist-high for balance. (This is called high guard.) They are unconsciously making sure they have their hands ready to break any falls that might occur, something we all do at any age when we're trying something new. Remember when you were learning how to roller skate, how you held your hands out to the side for balance and protection? Later, when you got the hang of it and relaxed, your arms naturally dropped to your sides when you skated. By the time your baby is 2 years old, her hands will have dropped to her sides, too, and her stride will be that of a confident grownup.

Your baby may be running now, too. The running style of a 15-month-old will not win her an Olympic medal.

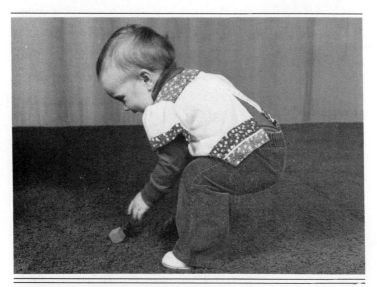

The 15-month-old can stoop to pick up a toy, then stand again. This is a sign of normal physical development.

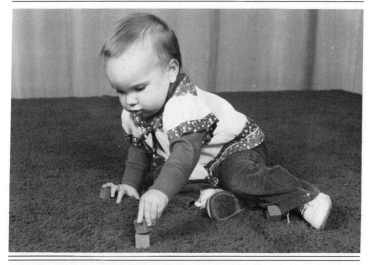

*At age 15 months, a toddler
can stack one block on top of another.*

Knees stiff, she probably resembles a tin solider rather than a long-distance runner, and she has trouble stopping and rounding corners. Like her walking, her running will mature. Meanwhile there is pure joy that she can now propel herself from one place to another, getting there in half the time and having twice as much fun. She can also walk upstairs with one hand held, and she has probably been creeping up-stairs by herself for several weeks.

From a standing position your toddler can stoop, pick up a toy, and then stand again. This stooped, or squatting, position is very typical of the 15-month-old. She can now throw a ball purposely when asked to do so. Throwing things (casting) just for the thrill of throwing them is about at its peak and may even have begun to subside.

Another accomplishment is that she can stack one cube or block on top of another to make a tower of two. If she's precocious, she may even be able to stack three blocks at a time. The practical implications of this are that many eager parents buy their children—especially their first

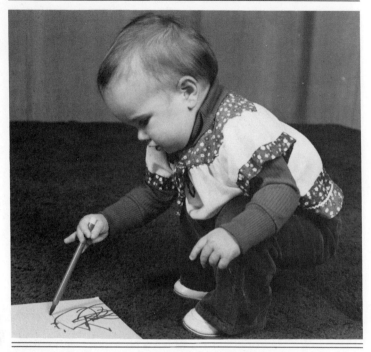

The 15-month-old can hold a pen or pencil and scribble spontaneously on a piece of paper. This is a sign of appropriate fine motor development.

children—building blocks many weeks before the youngsters have any notion of what to do with them. Your baby is now ready for building blocks.

A sign of progress in fine motor development is that your baby can hold a pencil and scribble spontaneously on a piece of paper. A pencil is not a safe plaything because of its sharp point, of course, so it is given to her by an examiner only as a screening test for development. But it won't be long before your child will enjoy crayons to scribble with on a regular basis.

Personal/Social Her table manners could almost qualify your offspring for a meal at a three-star restaurant. She can feed herself completely with only a moderate

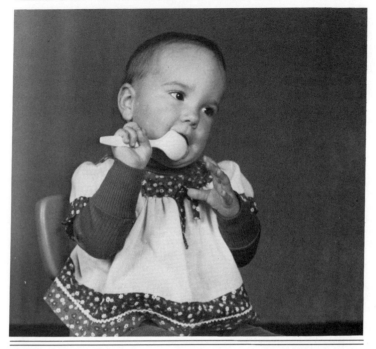

When using a spoon the 15-month-old tips it upside down just as it reaches her mouth. This is a normal reflex.

amount of spilling, using her fingers and a spoon. Although she is quite accomplished with a spoon, she still tips it upside down reflexively just as she gets it to her mouth. Some spilling results.

In nonverbal communication skills she has progressed from being able to point to instead of cry for things she wants (at one year) to being able to seek help actively from another person in order to perform a task. For example, she may bring you a wind-up toy that she is unable to wind herself, and it is quite clear that she wants you to do it for her. Or she may present you with a container that has a lid, indicating unmistakably that she wants you to remove the lid for her. Your child is also beginning to be interested in helping to dress herself, holding out her arms for sleeves, and so on. She is equally interested in undressing herself. She can manage to get her shoes off nicely and to tug at the toes of her socks as well.

Language Depending on which expert you believe, a 15-month-old has a vocabulary of (a) *Mama, Dada* plus three other words, (b) ditto plus ten other words, or (c) as many as eighteen other words! Suffice it to say that your child is certainly building her language skills with much help from you as you continue to talk to her, read to her, and tell her the names of objects and animals. There are

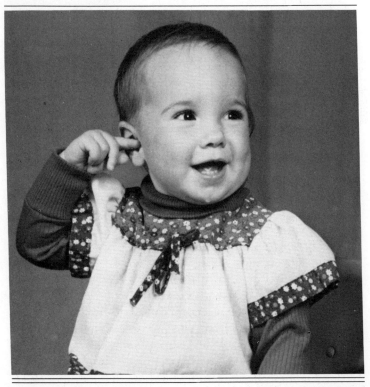

"Where is your ear?" gets a quick response from most 15-month-olds.

apocryphal tales of youngsters who speak not a word until they are 3 years old and then immediately begin to quote poetry. A more realistic expectation is that in the area of language, just as in every area of development, your toddler will proceed at her own pace according to her own genetic timetable. Whether she speaks one word or ten at this age, if she speaks it appropriately and distinctly, and if she appears to understand what is said to her, there is probably nothing to worry about. Check with your doctor, though, if you have doubts or questions about her speech development.

Fifteen months is an age when youngsters delight in pointing out body parts for any interested bystander. "Where is your ear?" and "Show me your nose" are a signal for most 15-month-olds to go into their act. Another endearing trait of children this age is the way they identify their peers as babies. "Baby," they say solemnly, pointing to a moppet exactly their own age or older. Most youngsters this age also have a word for "thank you," although it may be one of their own invention, such as "takoo" or "dank." The way they use it consistently and clearly indicates their intention of saying thanks.

NUTRITION

Be patient with your child's appetite. It helps to remember that you really don't feed a 15-month-old. She feeds herself. Some days her appetite may be gratifyingly large; others, infuriatingly small. Many days you have to be satisfied if just one of the three daily meals is a well-balanced one with "normal" helpings. There is usually no health risk related to this decline in appetite that many children experience beginning at about age 10 months and extending well into the second year of life. Your child is growing taller, but putting on less weight, so naturally she is thinner. This is normal. Any serious dropoff in height or weight percentiles will show up on the growth charts and records your doctor keeps for your baby. That's why babies are checked so frequently in the first two years, so that any danger signs can be picked up quickly and acted upon. It will help not to overwhelm your child with portions that are too large. Serve her small portions on small plates. Limit milk to 16 ounces a day, almost all of which should be taken by cup now. Either skim or whole milk is acceptable.

It is important to continue to offer the four basic food groups each day, and it is especially important during this period of possibly lessened appetite to either eliminate or severely limit the amount of sweets in the child's diet. These empty calories (of little or no nutritional value) can only further interfere with her appetite.

For safety's sake, a toddler should never be allowed to walk or run with lollipops or popsicles in her mouth, because the sticks could cause serious injury if she fell. And most toddlers fall often.

PARENT CONCERNS

Breath-holding   Breath-holding is an unnerving but common practice in some children in the first two years of life. It's a surefire attention-getter, and therein lies the problem. It tends to disappear as soon as it stops getting attention. So the first sign that your child is holding her breath is your signal to leave the room. With no one there to watch her turn blue and perhaps lose consciousness for a few seconds, there's little reward attached, and the behavior should end. If it doesn't, the doctor may be able to prescribe something that will help.

Fears   It is normal for children to be afraid of things from time to time, even things they've never been afraid of before. A child who has been perfectly contented with water experiences may suddenly become fearful of baths in a regular tub or swims in the neighborhood pool. Or a baby who has shown no previous fear of animals may inexplicably begin to be terrified of dogs or cats. Another common fear is of the vacuum cleaner and the roaring it makes. The 15-month-old may even show separation anxiety again. She may weep bitterly at being left with a babysitter, as she used to when she was younger.

Your patience and understanding will help. Don't try to

force the child to bathe in the tub, touch the vacuum cleaner, or make friends with the neighborhood Doberman. Instead, give her the opportunity to regain confidence in these areas slowly, always with you nearby, offering quiet encouragement. It can help to have the child bathe with an older sibling or even with you until she is ready to be alone in the tub again. Perhaps if she is allowed to turn the switch on the vacuum cleaner on and off herself (when she is ready to get that close) it will help. Acquiring a kitten or puppy for her may help with the animal fears. Everybody has fears. Only when they are so intense as to interfere with a normal life do they require professional counseling.

Hitting   Some parents wonder what to do when their babies hit them in frustration. And babies *do* strike out on occasion. Should the parents hit back? (*Gently*, of course.) Or should they ignore it? The answer is neither. Hitting back tells the child that hitting must be okay because her parents do it, that it is okay for big people to hit smaller people, and that her parents don't have control of their anger. Ignoring hitting, on the other hand, doesn't give enough reinforcement to the idea that hitting is not okay. A good response to hitting is time out, with the child sent to another room for a few minutes. Five minutes is long enough for a child this age.

Negativism   Although age 2 is the traditional time for children to reach their uncooperative stage, you may already be getting a sneak preview from your 15-month-old. It's a normal phase that will pass. It's a healthy expression of the independence that your baby strives for. You can help her through it by understanding that she wants and needs your support at the same time that she struggles to establish herself as somebody separate from you. You will continue to set boundaries for her behavior as always, but you should try to enforce them with your superior physical power as little as possible. The typical 15-month-old has moods and a temper that is easily aroused but (usually) quickly abates.

Sibling Rivalry   When she was a newborn, your baby may have been a threat to brothers or sisters, who had to learn to share your love and attention with her. Now they may be feeling even more threatened, for a 15-month-old gets more than just time and attention from her parents. She gets into everything with no respect for the property of elder siblings. Jealousy among siblings and a certain amount of rivalry and spatting are normal, but nobody should be allowed to get physically hurt.

Toilet Training   A few toddlers of this age may begin to notice when they're wet or soiled and try to bring it to their parents' attention. Such children may be ready for toilet training, but 18 months is a more likely time to begin.

REMINDERS

Safety Topics   Mr. Yuk. Your child may be old enough now to understand that Mr. Yuk, the antipoison sticker, means danger. Place the stickers on all toxic substances and be sure they are out of reach as well. This is probably one of the most dangerous periods of your child's life. She has plenty of physical skills but small sense of danger. It's a time when you not only need to watch her almost contstantly, but you also need to be sure you have taken all the childproofing precautions outlined in Chapter 3. Please take the time now to review that chapter.

Language Skills   With your help, your child is rapidly building her vocabulary. Continue to talk to her, read to her, *listen* to her, and explain things to her. Give her lots of picture books and old magazines.

Toys   Blocks. Things to put together and take apart. "Baby" puzzles with big wooden pieces. Push toys. Pull toys.

NEXT CHECKUP

Your baby will have her next checkup in three months, when she is 18 months old. Watch for the following milestones in development. Details are in the next chapter.

- Walks downstairs, one hand held
- Imitates housework

- Partially undresses self
- Increases vocabulary

RESOURCES

Mr. Yuk stickers are available free from your local pharmacy or poison-control center.

Briggs, Dorothy Corkille. **Your Child's Self-Esteem.** Garden City, N.Y.: Doubleday and Co., Inc., 1975.

Crary, Elizabeth. **Without Spanking or Spoiling.** Seattle: Parenting Press, 1979.

12
THE 18-MONTHS
CHECKUP

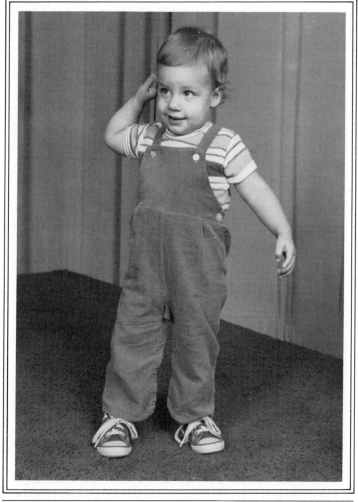

✓ CHECKLIST

18-MONTHS CHECKUP

Date _____

Procedures

_____ Weigh and measure

Weight _____

Percentile _____

Height _____

Percentile _____

Head circumference _____

_____ Discuss weight and height gains on growth charts with parents

_____ DTP & TOPV #4/immunizations against diphtheria, tetanus, pertussis (whooping cough), and polio

_____ Cover test for crossed eyes

_____ Hirschberg test for corneal reflections (crossed eyes)

_____ Discuss nutrition

_____ Ask about parent concerns

_____ Counsel on safety

PHYSICAL EXAMINATION*

Special attention to:

_____ Hearing

_____ Vision

_____ Developmental milestones (walks backward, runs, kicks ball)

_____ Gait

_____ Mouth for teeth

_____ Head for anterior fontanel

*The complete physical examination is described and illustrated in Chapter 4.

At the time of this examination, your child is due for his fourth set of shots in the DTP/TOPV series. These are to protect him against diphtheria, tetanus, pertussis (whooping cough), and polio. DTP is given as a single shot in the large muscle of the thigh. Polio vaccine is given by mouth as a few drops of fruit-flavored liquid. Your child will not need a booster shot for these diseases again until he is about 5 years old. (The American Academy of Pediatrics recommends that it be done between ages 4 and 6 years.)

If your child's reaction to the shots has been mild or absent in the past, there is no reason to suppose this one will be any different. If, however, there is swelling, soreness, hardness, or redness at the injection site, accompanied by fever or unusual fussiness, call the doctor's office to report it. Adverse reactions—especially serious ones—usually occur within the first 24 hours after immunization. Be sure to add these shots to a permanent record, such as the one provided at the back of this book. You are responsible for keeping your own and your children's medical records. Immunizations and the diseases they protect against are discussed in detail in Chapter 6.

THE PHYSICAL EXAMINATION

From the standpoint of cooperation, this examination could go either way. Fascinated by the doctor's tone of voice and his attentiveness as he talks the child through the examination, your 18-month-old may not protest in the

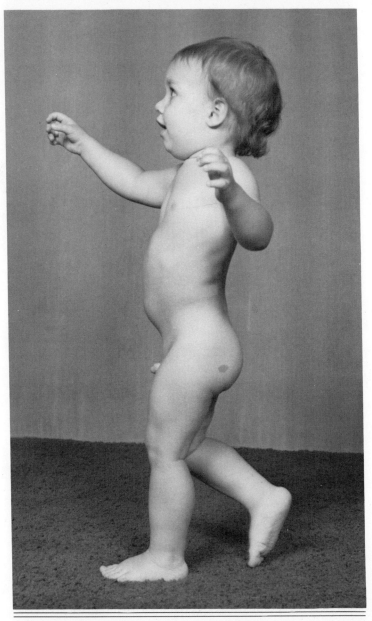

At age 18 months most children are slightly pot-bellied and swaybacked. This is normal.

slightest. On the other hand, if he has had a recent un-pleasantness in the doctor's office, such as stitches for a wound, he may wail the whole time. The examiner will have sympathy for and be prepared to deal with either reaction, so there is no reason for you to be embarrassed for your child or angry with him. If the examiner wants your help in quieting the child or holding him, she will let you know. To be afraid of a place where you've been hurt before—however good the intentions were—is not being naughty but intelligent.

The doctor will probably perform many, if not all, of the maneuvers described in Chapter 4. In examining the head, she will likely find that the anterior fontanel, the last remaining soft spot at the top of the child's head, has disappeared. This is because the bony plates in his skull have closed. It is possible for the soft spot to close later than 18 months, however—as late as 3 years of age in a normal child.

When your child stands, he has the distinctive posture normal for children of his age—slightly swaybacked and pot-bellied. Because he has recently been developing more muscles than fat, he is also thinner looking than when he was a baby. That, too, is normal.

In examining the mouth, the doctor will be interested in how many teeth your child has and what condition they're in. The "average" number of teeth for this age is 14 to 16, but it is normal for some children to have fewer than that. More than that is also normal, for some youngsters may already have a complete set of 20 by now. However many, there are enough teeth so that they need to be cleaned and cared for regularly. Care of these primary, or baby, teeth is extremely important. Only if they are kept clean and free of disease and decay will the permanent teeth that follow them be healthy. Brushing and flossing should be started now, if not sooner. See "Reminders," this chapter, for hints on how to do it.

The doctor may ask you if your child's eyes ever seem to cross. At this age that would indicate a problem. Two tests are performed to check for crossed eyes. One, the

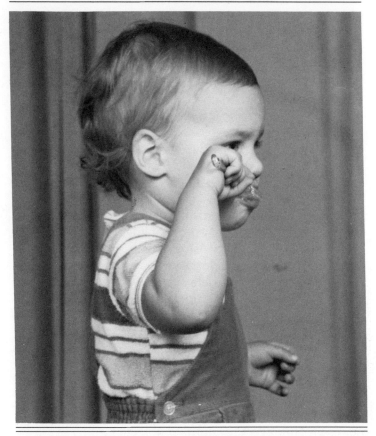

An 18-month-old interested in brushing his own teeth should be encouraged to do so, but he will need followup help to ensure thorough cleaning.

cover test, is frequently repeated at this checkup. The doctor covers one of the child's eyes with her hand and then uncovers it, observing the behavior of the eye carefully. She then repeats the test on the other eye. The second eye test frequently performed at age 18 months is the Hirschberg. Here the doctor holds a penlight at the child's eye level at a distance of about a foot. She looks at both eyes for the spot of light reflected from the corneas. In healthy eyes, both spots of light should show in exactly the same place on each eye.

As usual, the doctor will ask if your child appears to see and hear well. One clue to poor vision at this age might be a child who clings excessively to his parents. The child clings because he cannot move safely from place to place on his own. Such a child might also exhibit behavior mentioned in earlier chapters as well—straining to see, cocking the head to one side, covering or closing an eye, and holding objects very close to his eyes. A child who seems to fall more than usual may also have a vision problem. Report any of these signs to the doctor. She depends on your observations in such matters, since many clues to poor vision will not necessarily become apparent during the physical examination.

As for hearing, the most important indication of normal hearing at this age continues to be the development of normal speech. Though some words in your child's vocabularly will obviously be clearer than others, at least some of them should be clear. If he has a "language" of his own, which is perfectly normal at this age, it should be rich in tonal quality. That is, it should have high, low, and middle tones mixed so as to mimic real speech. The child should also be able to hear you when his back is turned toward you and you are speaking in a normal, or even a whispered, voice.

The last item in the examination, just before the shots, is usually to check the child's standing and walking, to be sure there is no toeing, either in or out, when he walks, that he is not knock-kneed, and that the arches and bones in his feet are developing normally.

MILESTONES IN DEVELOPMENT ± *
Motor/Physical
- Walks downstairs, one hand held
- Seats self in adult chair

*The plus-or-minus sign indicates that your child may very well reach developmental milestones earlier or later than what is indicated here as "average." There is a wide range of normal in child development.

- Walks backwards
- Runs well
- Runs into ball (not a true kick)

Personal/Social
- Imitates housework
- Interested in dressing and undressing self
- Gets spoon to mouth right-side-up
- Drinks well from cup

Language/Communication
- Vocabulary of 3 to 29 words (some not spoken too clearly but many intelligible)
- Combines two to three words ("all gone")
- Combines two ideas ("baby bed, Daddy go")
- Points to two to four body parts
- Follows two simple commands at once ("Give cup to Mother.")
- Points to pictures in book ("Where's the dog?")

Progress at age 18 months in every area of development can be summed up nicely as the fine art of doing two things at once. Until now your toddler has mastered things one at a time. Now, however, he is perfecting them *two* at a time, and it is very exciting to watch. He can walk and carry a toy, walk and push a toy, or creep and push a toy. He can walk and pull a toy. (He can even walk backwards and pull a toy.) He can combine two words and two ideas. And he can obey two commands at once.

Motor/Physical   At 15 months, toddlers walk upstairs with one hand held. At 18 months they progress to the more difficult task of walking downstairs with one hand held. A few even climb up and down stairs on their own, holding on to the railing for support. The 18-month-old walks and runs well and falls little, though his knees are still stiff. About 75 percent of youngsters this age can walk backward as well as forward if they are shown how to do it. They also try to kick. Given a large ball to play with, they imitate kicking by running toward the ball and bumping it. But there is no true kick yet.

At this age your child can probably climb into a big

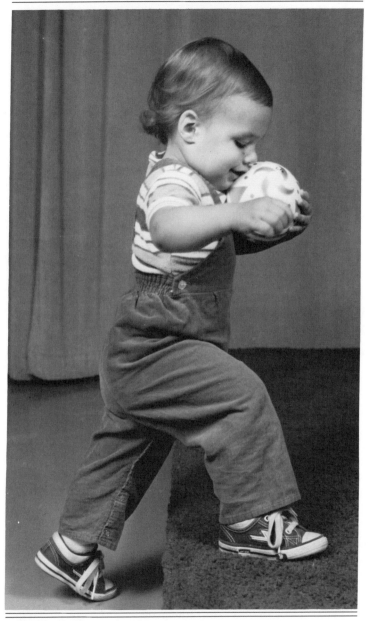

*Doing two things at a time
comes naturally for the 18-month-old.*

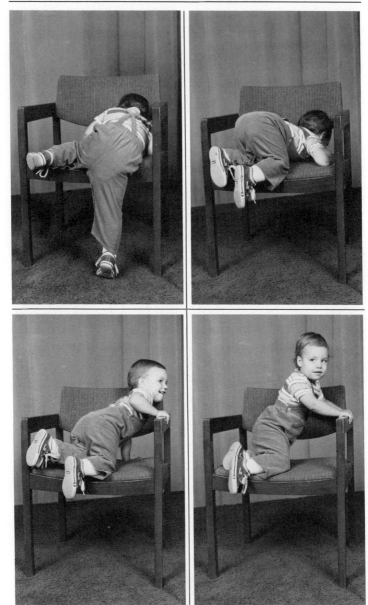

*At age 18 months a child can climb easily into
an adult chair, a sign of normal physical development.*

chair and seat himself in it quite gracefully. He can sit in a small chair by backing into it, adult fashion, and would very much enjoy a small chair of his own now if he doesn't already have one. Fine motor skills include his being able to stack three or four blocks on top of one another and being able to turn the pages of a book or magazine by himself, two or three pages at a time.

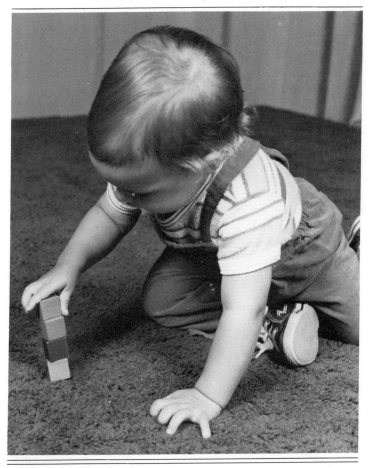

The fine motor skills of an 18-month-old include stacking three or flour blocks.

Personal/Social   The typical 18-month-old imitates the household tasks he sees his parents do—mopping, sweeping, dusting, hammering, and mowing the lawn. It is an age at which he will enjoy having toy tool sets, a child-size broom, and unbreakable toy dishes. He values equally the tasks he observes both parents do and has fun with them all. He makes no distinction between hugging a doll, hammering a peg, or setting the table. This needn't worry you.

The 18-month-old is very interested in dressing and undressing himself. He can be quite skilled at taking off his shoes, socks, and, with a little help from you, most of his clothes. He's much better at taking them off than he is in putting them back on, however. He has a sense of how things should look when they're done right, so instead of slapping a cowboy hat haphazardly on his head, he gets it on properly.

He has reached an important landmark in feeding himself with a spoon. Until now he has rotated the spoon just as it reached his mouth, tipping it upside down and spilling some of its contents. He had no control over that; it was a kind of reflex that all youngsters have when first learning to manage a spoon. Now he can get the spoon to his mouth right-side-up, food intact. He is also very accomplished with his cup. He can pick it up, drink from it, and put it back on his tray neatly, spilling little. Gone (almost) are the wild arcs in the air with the cup and the generous puddles on the floor under his high chair.

Language/Communication   Toddlers of 18 months may have a vocabulary of up to 29 words, but most are able to say at least three to five words in addition to *Mama* and *Dada*. Ten words is average. Although some of the words in his vocabulary may not be spoken too clearly, most are intelligible and can be understood by family members. He knows how to ask for more, and he knows how to ask for foods specifically, such as *cookie* or *drink*. Young children seem to know that it is far better to be able to be specific with their needs, so most prefer, if they are able, to ask for a cookie rather than to grunt and point at one. If your child is

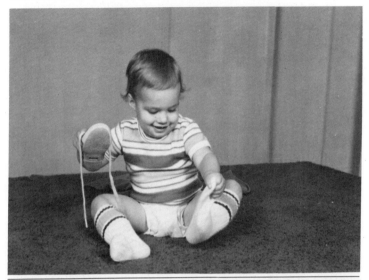

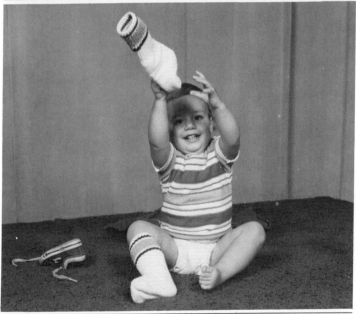

Interested in dressing and undressing himself, the 18-month-old is particularly skilled at taking off his shoes and socks.

still mostly grunting and pointing, mention it to the doctor at this checkup. There is probably nothing to worry about, but your doctor may want to make a note of it and follow it up at the next exam.

The "average" 18-month-old can combine two words. *All gone* and *oh dear* are favorite combinations. He can also combine two ideas. When he says "Baby bed" or "Daddy gone," he is combining two ideas as well as two words. That is a real milestone in his speech development. He can follow two simple commands at the same time, too, such as "Give the cup to Mother" or "Throw the ball to Dad."

He can point to two to four (and possibly more) body parts and enjoys being asked where his nose, ear, mouth, and bellybutton are. He will cheerfully point them out to anyone who's interested. He can also point out specific animals and objects in a picture book and enjoys being asked, "Where's the dog?" or "Show me the ball." He is interested in picture books now for longer periods of time before becoming bored with them.

Children who live in homes where two languages are spoken are somewhat slower to acquire language skills in the beginning. It's not hard to understand why it is twice as difficult for the bilingual youngster to sort things out. He has to master two words for each object and keep them separate. He has twice as much information to absorb, store, and use. Once past this first hurdle, though, bilingual children are able to catch up with their age group in language skills, usually by the time they reach school age.

NUTRITION

By now your child should have made the transition from baby foods to table foods, and he should be able to participate in family mealtimes, eating what everybody else eats, with a few exceptions. There are still foods that should be withheld because of the danger of inhaling (aspirating) them and choking on them. These include raw carrots, celery, and apples; nuts (even those baked into cakes and cookies); popcorn, and raisins. Remember, too, that it is very dangerous for a child to walk or run with a popsicle or lollipop (sucker) in his mouth. Sour balls and other small, suckable candies are also very dangerous. It is best to avoid all these foods for at least the first three years of life and possibly longer.

Give your child the opportunity now to feed himself entirely with a spoon and cup. His abilities with both are good to excellent, although he still sometimes looks upon mealtimes as an opportunity for messy play. Limit sweets. The damage they do to teeth can be somewhat lessened if you allow them to be eaten once a day—dessert after dinner, for example—and then clean the child's teeth immediately afterward.

Offer servings from each of the four basic food groups each day—dairy products, grains, fruits and vegetables, meat and fish without bones. Milk should be restricted to 16 ounces a day, and table foods are suitable at every meal. The 18-month-old may have an erratic appetite and may also have developed definite likes and dislikes in foods. He may become passionate for some things at the exclusion of others. He can't get enough mashed potatoes for a month, for example, then won't touch them for another month. Don't make a battle out of it; just switch to bread or pasta for a while.

Although many toddlers experience a normal reduction in appetite in their second year, some do not. Your toddler will not necessarily become a picky eater, but here are some things to think about if he does. You have control over what kind of food he eats, but not how much. In choosing foods for him, you'll be doing him a great favor and instilling good nutritional habits that will last a lifetime if you restrict sweets and salt and introduce him to the pleasures of fresh fruits, fruit juices, and vegetables as snack foods. Again, you control the choice of foods but not the amount eaten.

When you're 18 months old, almost everything is more interesting than taking time to eat. A grownup's mealtimes, after all, are cultural to some extent, and they are scheduled at rigid hours as well. The child's desire for meals, on the other hand, is strictly related to hunger. It is only reasonable to expect that some days the child's hunger and the parents' scheduled mealtimes will not match. As a result, there will be meals untouched, meals played with, and meals completely eaten. Before you look for professional help, take a look at the child's eating behavior over a three- or four-day period for volume. Viewed from that perspective, the highs and lows smooth out. There is professional help available, of course, when it is truly needed, and your doctor will be able to make recommendations. Meanwhile, there are a lot more important things for you and your toddler to disagree about than a clean plate. And finally, however quirky his appetite, his body is simply not going to let him starve.

PARENT CONCERNS

(These are only some of the concerns parents have at this checkup. Be sure you have yours written down to discuss with the doctor.)

Discipline The whys and hows of discipline are much easier to talk about than they are to act upon. It helps, though, to understand why children need discipline in their lives. Setting boundaries for them is a reassuring sign of your love and concern. It is a stepping stone to the time when they can set their own boundaries. All discipline is, really, is helping your child to reach self-discipline.

At about 18 months of age—sometimes a little earlier or later—the child makes a big push to establish his independence from you. This is natural and to be encouraged, for it is something he needs to do. He will not make such a marked separation effort again until he is an adolescent. His behavior during this fledgling independence may become negative, and he may begin to test severely the limits you've set on his behavior. You must decide what those limits are, remembering that you should try to be fair and reasonable and set limits that are both enforceable and worth enforcing. Hitting, biting, and kicking are good examples of behavior you might reasonably find unacceptable. Having set the limits, you need only follow up on them consistently with the patience of a saint.

Acting on limits consistently and patiently is more difficult by far than setting them. If hitting is not okay one day, it is not okay any day. So each time there is hitting, there must be a patient, nonviolent response from you, such as time out for a few minutes. Your goal should also be to punish without anger. That doesn't mean you should never get angry, just that you shouldn't *act* in anger. Timing is also important. The time-out punishment should occur as soon as the transgression occurs. You should also explain to the child briefly and clearly why he's having time out.

Thumbsucking   Thumbsucking, discussed more fully in Chapter 7, peaks at age 18 months. It is normal behavior.

Toilet Training.   Your child may be ready for toilet training. Depending on the signals you get from him, any time between now and age 2 is a good time to begin. He is ready when he can signal his needs before he needs to go or when he comes to be cleaned up afterward. The switch from diapers to training pants is an excellent incentive for most children.

Bladder control is often easier to accomplish with youngsters than bowel control. As their urinary bladders mature, children begin to be dry for increasingly long periods, and they quickly catch on to telling you when they want to urinate. Training for bowel movements is more difficult for some children. It's important not to apply too much pressure or make too much of an issue of it, for it could result in the child's deliberately withholding bowel movements (encopresis). This condition is very difficult to deal with once it has been established.

If there is resistance to toilet training, it is wise to postpone it for a while. Like the dinner table, the potty should not become a battleground. Toilet training as late as the third year is normal (although some parents find it unacceptably late). When toilet training is in progress, expect accidents. They will certainly happen in the beginning. Also, if you are trying to establish toilet training to coincide with the birth of another child, you may find that your youngster loses ground with his toilet training when the new baby is brought home.

REMINDERS

Safety Topics   Falls, poisonings, burns, choking, drowning, automobile accidents. These continue to be the biggest threat to your child's good health. Ways to make your home and car safer are discussed in Chapter 3.

Tooth Care   An 18-month-old interested in brushing his own teeth should be encouraged to do so, but he will need follow-up help to ensure thorough cleaning. When you brush your child's teeth, have him in a comfortable position, such as lying semireclined with his head in your lap. Use a small brush with soft bristles that are cut straight across. Brush all surfaces of each tooth carefully.

Use dental floss to clean between teeth. Holding it taut with thumbs and forefingers about an inch apart, insert the floss gently between the teeth, using an up-and-down motion. Be careful not to use a brisk, sawing motion that could injure the gums. Use a new section of floss for each space between teeth. You'll need a piece about 18 inches long. The child's teeth should be brushed after every meal. They should be especially carefully brushed and flossed before bedtime to prevent plaque from forming and doing damage during sleeping hours.

Toys   Push and pull toys. Child-size mops and brooms and unbreakable toy dishes. Hammering benches, empty boxes, doll carriages, small wagons. Retail store catalogs. This is a good age for a child to have a small chair of his own. Let him shop for it with you, so that together you can find one that is just right.

NEXT CHECKUP

Your child's next checkup will be in six months, when he is 2 years old. It will be helpful if you take him to that examination in a pair of old shoes so that the doctor can examine them for normal wear patterns.

Between now and the next checkup, look for the following milestones in development.

- Kicks ball by swinging leg
- Turns doorknobs, unscrews lids (Be sure all medicines are out of reach, as well as cleaning agents and other poisonous substances.)
- Asks to go potty at least some of the time
- Increases his vocabulary

13
THE 2-YEAR
CHECKUP

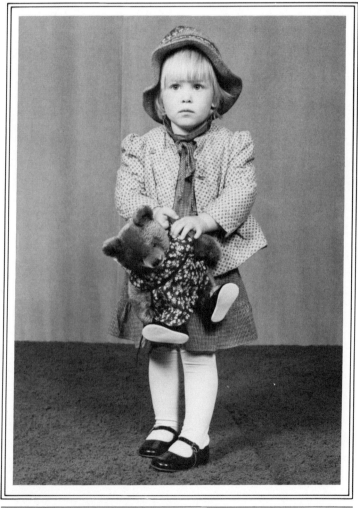

✓ CHECKLIST

2-YEAR CHECKUP

Date _____

Procedures

_____ Weigh and measure

Weight _____

Percentile _____

Height _____

Percentile _____

Head circumference _____

_____ Discuss weight and height gains on growth charts with parents

_____ Cover test for crossed eyes

_____ Hematocrit (Hct)/Hemoglobin (Hgb) blood test (optional)

_____ Hirschberg test for corneal response to light (crossed eyes)

_____ Blood pressure (optional)

_____ Tuberculosis test (optional)

_____ Urinalysis (optional)

_____ Discuss nutrition

_____ Ask about parent concerns

_____ Counsel on safety and behavior

PHYSICAL EXAMINATION*

Special attention to:

_____ Hearing and speech

_____ Gait

_____ Developmental milestones (walks, runs, walks up and down stairs by self)

_____ Teeth and teeth care

*The complete physical examination is discussed and illustrated in Chapter 4.

Weight and height statistics at this checkup are meaningful, for by now the average 2-year-old has quadrupled her birthweight and increased her birth length by 70 percent. If she weighed 8 pounds at birth and was 20 inches long, she will now weigh about 32 pounds and be about 34 inches tall. You can even estimate how tall she will be when she grows up. Two-year-olds are *approximately* half as tall as they will be when they are fully grown. A 34-inch-tall 2-year-old, then, would be about 5 feet 8 inches tall at maturity. Remember, though, that these are only rough guidelines, not exact predictions.

The cover and Hirschberg eye tests, both described in previous chapters, are commonly repeated at the 2-year checkup. There are two other procedures, both optional, that might also be performed at age 2 years. One is a urine test; the other is measurement of the child's blood pressure.

Urine tests are designed to detect bacteria, blood, sugar, and protein in the urine. Since normal urine is sterile, it should contain none of those things (except that girls' urine normally contains small amounts of bacteria). Their presence indicates either infection or disease and suggests that further investigation and perhaps treatment are necessary.

Urinalysis includes placing into a urine specimen a specially treated dipstick that shows the presence of protein and sugar. Then the specimen is centrifuged (spun at high speed) and studied under a microscope to detect any foreign cells or bacteria. A second kind of urine test is called urine culture. It involves growing bacteria from the urine specimen in a special culture in order to identify the exact strain of invading bacteria.

Some doctors believe, however, that routine screening programs for urinary-tract infections in all their patients is expensive and ineffective. They feel it is more productive to investigate individually those children who either have a history of infection or who show some signs of it. Signs and symptoms of urinary tract infection include frequency, urgency, painful urination, dribbling, foul-smelling urine, bloody or cloudy urine, and wetting in a child who was previously trained and dry. There may also be fever, irritability, and stomach pains. Any of these signs or symptoms should be reported right away to the doctor for further evaluation. It is important to begin treatment of urinary-tract infections immediately. Although some are self-limiting—meaning they get better by themselves—others are not and can spread to the kidneys, where permanent damage can occur.

Except in early infancy, urinary-tract infections are more common in girls than boys. Anatomy has a great deal to do with this. A girl's urethra (the tube between the bladder and the surface) is shorter and closer to the surface than that of a boy, so that foreign bacteria have easier entrance and a shorter distance to travel. That's why girls should be cleaned from front to back in the genital area. Otherwise bacteria from bowel movements can easily invade the urinary tract. Cotton underpants are healthier for youngsters than nylon ones, which trap moisture and promote the growth of bacteria.

Although taking the blood pressure is usually included in the physical examination beginning at age 3 years, it is sometimes done as early as age 2. Uncommon in children of this age, high blood pressure (hypertension) is most likely an indication of either kidney disease or abnormalities in the blood vessels that lead from the heart.

Blood pressure is a measure of blood flow from the heart. Two readings are taken. The first is done when the

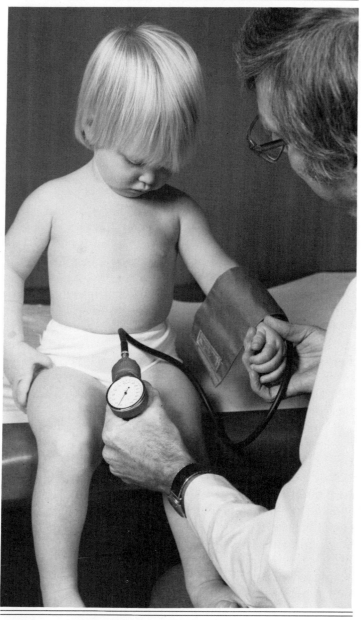

*Taking the blood pressure is
sometimes part of the 2-year checkup.*

heart squeezes down and the blood flows the fastest through the body. This is called systolic pressure. The second reading is taken when the heart relaxes and the flow of blood slows. It is diastolic pressure. To take blood pressure, an instrument is used called a sphygmomanometer, which consists of a cloth arm cuff, a rubber-bulb syringe that pumps air into the cuff, and a pressure gauge much like the one on a pressure cooker.

The doctor wraps the cuff around the child's upper right arm and pumps air into the cuff until blood flow in the arm is stopped. Then he releases the air slowly, listening at the same time with the stethoscope to a spot just above the crook of the arm, where the brachial artery is located. As air is released, he hears a sharp banging noise that coincides with the pulse and signifies that blood is flowing again. The point at which the sounds are first heard represents the fast part of the blood pressure reading, the systolic pressure. The point at which sounds disappear is taken as the second part of the blood pressure reading, the diastolic. Blood pressure is expressed as a fraction. The top number represents systolic pressure (appearance of sound); the bottom, diastolic (disappearance of sound). Normal blood pressure for children between the ages of one and 4 years is about 90/60, with the systolic ranging from 35 to 100 and the diastolic from 50 to 70.

Another way to measure blood pressure in children younger than age 3 years is called the flush method. With this method, the blood is squeezed briefly from a hand or a foot by wrapping it tightly. Pressure is then pumped up in the blood pressure cuff, which has been attached to a wrist or ankle rather than to the usual position on the upper arm. Then the hand (or foot) is unwrapped, and the cuff pressure slowly released. A reading is taken when the extremity flushes red, indicating the point at which blood flow is restored. With this method there is only one reading, and the figure represents the mean, or average, blood pressure, halfway between the systolic and diastolic pressures.

By any method, obtaining a child's blood pressure is tricky and difficult, and the examiner may have to repeat the procedure once or twice to be sure of his results. Three determinations are not unusual and are, in fact, recommended.

A tuberculosis test will be performed at this checkup if your child is in a high-risk population group (where the incidence of the disease is greater than 1 percent). Depending on her diet, a blood test—either a hematocrit or a hemoglobin—may be performed to check for iron deficiency anemia. It will probably not be done if she is eating three well-balanced meals a day.

Examination of the mouth may reveal as many as 20 teeth. All 20 baby teeth are commonly in place by age 2 years, although some youngsters will, of course, have fewer. The full 20 include four (two on top, two on bottom from the center to the side) of each of the following: central

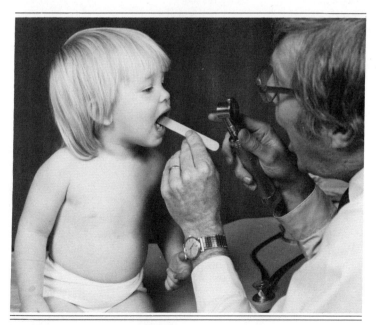

Examination of the mouth may reveal as many as 20 teeth. All 20 baby teeth are commonly in place by age 2 years.

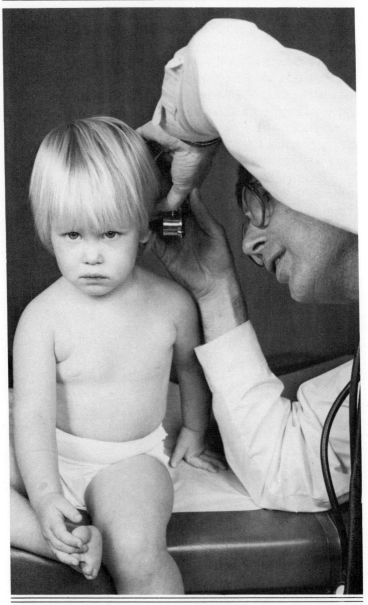

*Ears are checked for disease, infection,
and occasionally for beans, erasers, and other
objects placed there by the 2-year-old.*

incisors, lateral incisors, canines, first molars, and second molars.

Be very glad if there are good-sized gaps between each of your 2-year-old's teeth, for if there are not, your future orthodontist bills will almost certainly be high. Consider that these 20 baby teeth will be replaced by 32 bigger, permanent ones. In order for there to be room for them, the 20 baby teeth must have spaces in between, even allowing for the fact that the child's jaw will grow some between now and age 6, when her permanent teeth begin to come in.

Although eyes and ears are checked at each exam, vision and hearing are somewhat more difficult to assess. Eye examination with the ophthalmoscope will show whether there is any tumor or obstruction. Examination with the penlight will confirm that the pupils react properly to light (by reducing in size) and will rule out crossed eyes if the reflections from the corneas appear at the same spot on each eye. The cover test will also identify crossed or wandering eyes. But how well the child really sees cannot be determined for about one year, when she is old enough to take an eye test.

Similarly, ears can be checked for obstructions like the beans and erasers that sometimes find their way into the ear canal. They can also be checked for disease and infection. But how well your child really hears cannot be determined with any real accuracy until she is older. In the meantime, her speech is an excellent indication of her hearing ability. She should have a vocabulary of at least 50 words, many of which should be spoken clearly.

MILESTONES IN DEVELOPMENT ±*

Motor/Physical
• Walks well, walks backward
• Runs well, knees no longer stiff
• Walks up and down stairs by self, holding rail

---

*The plus-or-minus sign indicates that your child may very well reach developmental milestones earlier or later than what is indicated here as "average." There is a wide range of normal in child development.

- Jumps with both feet off floor
- Kicks ball by swinging leg
- Builds tower of up to seven blocks
- Turns doorknob, unscrews lids

Personal/Social
- Feeds self neatly, begins to use fork
- Drinks all fluids from cup
- Asks to go potty at least some of the time
- Helps with simple household tasks
- Dresses self partly, undresses self almost completely
- Washes and dries hands
- Plays near, but not with, other children

Language/Communication
- Talks a lot; vocabulary of 50+ words
- Uses two- to four-word sentences
- Uses *I, you, me, mine* correctly
- Uses plurals correctly
- Explains what's happening in picture book
- Names one to three items in picture book
- Turns book pages one at a time
- Describes experiences as they happen ("I kick ball")
- Names one body part

To be in a room full of 2-year-olds is to observe firsthand the whole range of human development. Some children are in diapers. Others, toilet trained, wear training pants. Some speak clearly in remarkably lengthy sentences, some talk baby talk, and some have little to say. Some cling to their mothers out of shyness; others race about the room exploring on their own. A few share the toys that have been made available to them. Most do not. But the most remarkable thing is that they are all *normal, healthy 2-year-olds* proceeding at their own pace.

Motor/Physical   The 2-year-old walks with great confidence, arms comfortably at her side like a grownup. As a toddler she held her arms waist-high for balance and as a buffer against falling. When she runs, her knees are no longer stiff, and she has lost that tin-soldier look. She can walk up and down stairs by herself, holding on to the rail.

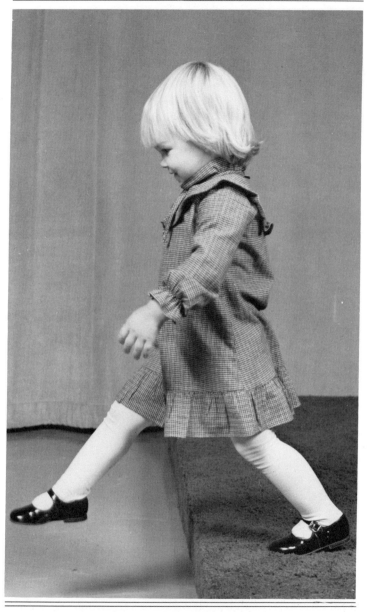

The 2-year-old walks with great confidence,
arms comfortably at her side like a grownup.

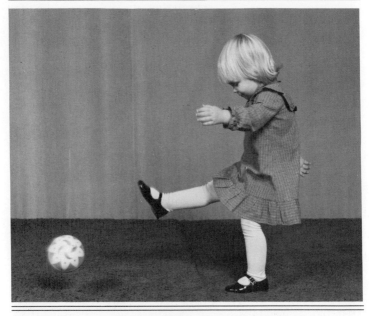

*The 2-year-old has a true kick, drawing back her
leg purposefully rather than just running into the ball.*

She doesn't mount the steps in adult fashion, though.
Instead, she steps up with one foot, then brings her other
foot up to the same step before mounting the next one. She
comes back down the same way, two feet planted before
moving on to the next step.

Most 2-year-olds can jump up with both feet off the
floor, something they do almost unconsciously when excited. They can also jump down with both feet from a low
height, such as the bottom step of a stairway. Kicking, too,
is a recent accomplishment. Whereas younger children run
into a ball to make it move, 2-year-olds draw back their legs
and kick the ball purposefully.

Your 2-year-old's manual dexterity is increasing as
well. She can build a tower of up to seven blocks, copy a
straight line or a circle with pencil and paper, and put small
things into containers. She can also turn doorknobs and

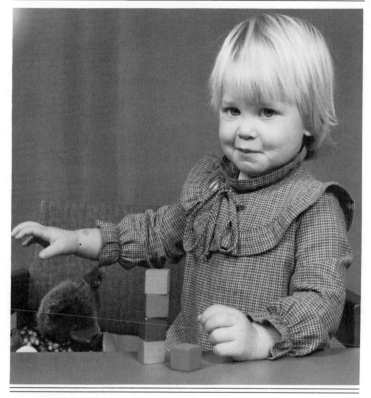

*The 2-year-old can build a
tower of from four to seven blocks.*

unscrew the lids on jars, bottles, and other containers. These last two accomplishments increase her risk of injury and accidental poisoning. Be sure that doors that lead to danger—such as those at the top of steep, unlighted basement stairs—are kept locked or bolted. The danger from her being able to easily manipulate containers is clear. It increases tremendously the risk of accidental poisoning. Be sure all prescription medications and cleaning preparations are in childproof containers and stored, either locked up or well out of reach. Use Mr. Yuk stickers generously.

Personal/Social   Most 2-year-olds feed themselves

neatly when they want to, and many are ready to begin to use a fork. They are skilled at drinking from a cup, so that weighted cups with lids are no longer necessary. All their fluids should be taken by cup now. No more bottles.

Although there may still be frequent accidents, most 2-year-olds ask to go potty at least some of the time. Typically they are more resistant to bowel than to bladder training.

Two-year-olds can help with simple household tasks such as folding laundry and putting toys away. (The laundry will have to be refolded later, but the child loves to help.) Some say they can be counted on to carry good china plates from one place to another, but paper plates might be a better idea for a while longer.

If dressing is fun for a 2-year-old, undressing is even more fun, and a naked 2-year-old is not an uncommon sight. Although she can only partly dress herself, she can

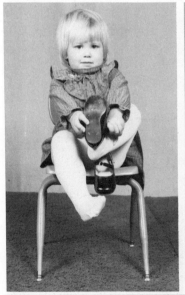
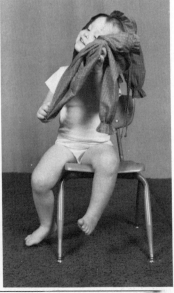

Undressing is great fun for a 2-year-old.

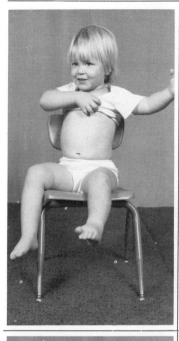
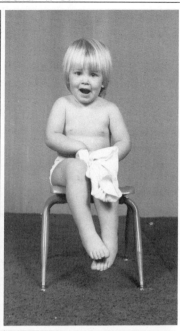
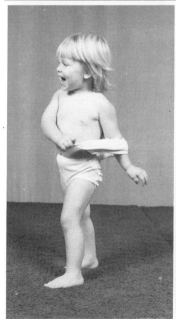
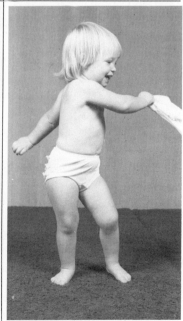

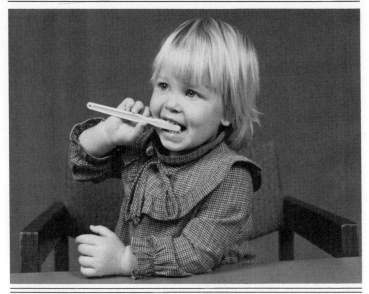

Most 2-year-olds can hold a toothbrush properly and are capable of performing the initial part of their daily brushing.

completely undress herself. When dressing, she still needs help with sleeves, zippers, buttons, and tying her shoes. About half of all children age 2 can wash and dry their own hands with supervision. Many can hold a toothbrush properly and should be permitted to do at least the preliminary part of daily teeth cleaning.

Two-year-olds play alongside other children, but they don't really play *with* them. Although it is too early for cooperative play, there are still many benefits from exposing your child to other children at this age. Children learn a great deal from each other by watching.

Language/Communication Most 2-year-olds talk a lot. You might even say they never seem to shut up. But there are still plenty of silent types who have little to say. The "average" 2-year-old has a vocabulary of more than 50 words (in some cases many more than 50) and can put

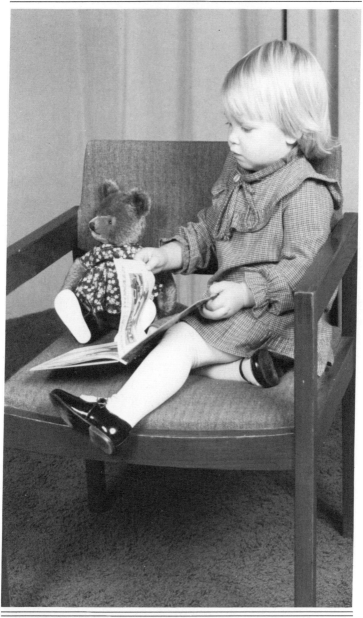

*A 2-year-old can turn book pages one at a time,
a sign of normal physical development.*

three words together. So if you aren't hearing at least a dozen words spoken clearly and appropriately by your 2-year-old, mention it to the doctor at this checkup. Also, your child should just about have given up jargon and baby talk except for those baby words that you yourself reinforce by using them deliberately in conversation with her.

Two-year-olds use *I, you, me* and *mine* correctly, and they also speak in sentences. The sentences may be anywhere from two to four or more words in length, but being able to put at least two or three words together at this age is considered to be an important sign of normal speech development. It is, in turn, an encouraging sign of normal hearing.

About half of all 2-year-olds use plurals correctly and can explain what's happening in a picture book. They can correctly identify one horse as "horsie" and two as "horsies." They are also able to explain what the horses are doing ("Horsie run") and to turn the book pages one at a time. Not only can they describe what is happening in a picture book, but they can describe their own and others' experiences as they happen as well—"Daddy go" or "I kick ball."

As a toddler, your child could point to a number of body parts. Now she can actually name at least one. Touch her nose, for instance, and ask her what it is, and the answer will be sure and quick—"NOSE!"

NUTRITION

The nutrition story is the same one you've been hearing for several months. Concerning appetite and food consumption, there are hungry days and not-so-hungry, finished meals and unfinished meals. It is encouraging to remember that you can at least control the foods that are served, even if you can't control the amount that is eaten. Offer small portions of a variety of nutritious foods from the four food groups—dairy, cereal and grain, fruit and vegetable, meat and fish without bones. Offer snacks that are low in sugar. If your child is a picky eater, no snacks at all or a few ounces of fruit juice might be a better idea. If your child is not a picky eater, the doctor will probably not prescribe supplementary vitamins for her. Vitamins are usually not prescribed if a child is eating well.

Completely weaned from bottle or breast to cup, a 2-year-old should be able to eat table foods at every meal. Only those foods that are dangerous and can cause choking should be withheld—nuts, popcorn, raisins, raw celery, and carrots. At age 2 years the size of portions increases slightly from what they were at age one. Dairy products increase from ½ cup to ¾ cup and citrus fruits from ⅓ to ½ cup per serving. Vegetables increase from 2 to 3 tablespoons at each serving. In the cereal and grain group, cereal portions increase from ¼ to ⅓ cup and bread portions from a half slice to a whole slice per serving. Meat and the protein foods stay the same—one egg per serving and

SIZE OF APPROXIMATE DAILY SERVINGS

Food Group	Age One	Age Two
Milk and dairy group (4 servings) cheese, cottage cheese, yogurt	½ cup	½–¾ cup
Meat group (3 + servings)		
eggs	1	1
lean meat, fish, poultry	2 Tbsp	2 Tbsp
peanut butter*		1 Tbsp
Fruits and vegetables (4 or more servings)		
Vitamin C source Citrus and other fruits, berries, tomatoes, cabbage, and cantaloupe	⅓ cup	½ cup
Others	2 Tbsp	3 Tbsp
Grain group (4 or more servings) bread	½ slice	1 slice
ready-to-eat cereals	½ ounce	¾ ounce
cooked cereal, macaroni, spaghetti	¼ cup	½ cup

*Not to be eaten by the spoonful because of the danger of choking.
Adapted from *Textbook of Pediatrics,* ed. Waldo E. Nelson, M.D., 11th ed.: 147.

about 2 tablespoons of well-chopped meat, fish, or poultry per serving. Seeing the food chart on the previous page. Keep in mind that these are only estimates. Some children regularly eat more or less than these amounts and still maintain a normal rate of growth.

PARENT CONCERNS

(These are only some of the concerns parents have at this checkup. Be sure you have yours written down to discuss with the doctor.)

Negativism Two-year-olds are easy to recognize. They're the ones who answer "no," firmly, to any question or request. Typically, they're negative and somewhat uncooperative. They may obey simple commands, but usually they're imperious and domineering. Indirect approaches work better with them than anything else. If your 2-year-old is not negative, congratulate yourself on your good fortune, but if she is, brace yourself for a period of patience, firmness and understanding.

Sharing It's not the nature of a 2-year-old to share, not willingly, at least. In a room full of 2-year-olds, some snatching goes on between children, but few give up what's theirs without protest. This is to be expected. Although you probably want to encourage sharing in your child, remember that even adult sharing is selective. When was the last time you shared your favorite perfume or your brand-new car with your neighbors? The truth is that none of us shares indiscriminately and it is unreasonable to expect our children to do so.

The 2-year-old has, after all, only recently developed the words for *me* and *mine.* The concept they stand for is powerful, and parents should be sensitive to when the child should be encouraged to share and when she needs some sympathy for something that got yanked out of her hand.

Temper Tantrums Everybody knows about the "terrible two's" and that 2-year-olds have tantrums. In fact, some do and some don't. Don't assume your child will have them, but if she does, it isn't because she's naughty and uncooperative but because she's trying to gain control of some small part of her environment. Two-year-olds have to learn to express the anger and frustration they feel because their desires don't yet match their skills or the amount of power they have. Your 2-year-old would like to control the number of cookies she eats each day. She would like to make her own decisions about whether or not she'll nap and what time she goes to bed. These decisions, however, are all made for her by somebody else, just as they have been all her life. Naturally she gets frustrated sometimes, and the result of her frustration can be tantrums.

Ignore tantrums whenever possible. When a tantrum takes place in a crowded supermarket, this can be the hardest possible advice to follow. It's not easy to ignore a screaming bundle of rage in your shopping cart. Tantrums at home are somewhat easier to deal with because you can give the child time out by herself in another room to get control of herself. Or you can leave the room yourself, denying the child an audience for her anger. In that way you won't be reinforcing her out-of-control behavior.

There is really no way to reason with or console a child in the grip of a fullblown tantrum. Such a child has to be given time out for as long as it takes her to quiet down. Never ridicule her, and try not to be angry with her. When she has regained control, it will help to go to her immediately and tell her how happy you are that she is feeling better about things. In that way you reward the good behavior and ignore the bad.

Sleep Disturbances   Sleep disturbances can occur at any time, beginning in infancy and extending throughout childhood. Some babies have more trouble than others from the very beginning in establishing sleep patterns that match those of their parents. Other infants seem to be light sleepers or even to require less sleep than average. Even children who usually sleep well occasionally have bad dreams or wake up in the middle of the night and feel panic they don't understand. Such children may need to be comforted and held for a few minutes.

It is natural for active children to be reluctant to give up the day and give in to sleep. So they stall, complain, ask repeatedly for drinks of water, and invent excuses to get out of bed. Sometimes it helps to have a quiet time with them just before bedtime, reading a favorite story or talking about the events of the day. It's not a good idea to engage in wrestling matches or other stimulating activity just before bedtime because the child gets too worked up to sleep.

Toilet Training   Most 2-year-olds are able and willing at least part of the time to tell their parents they need to use the toilet. Reward for such behavior should be lavish. Praise the child. In her presence tell other family members about her accomplishment. Accidents will happen, of course, but your attitude toward them should be casual.

REMINDERS

Safety Topics   Safe play outdoors. See Chapter 3.

Dental Care   By now your child ought to be at least partially responsible for her own teeth. She can brush them herself, although you will want to complete the job to be sure it is done thoroughly. She can also use toothpaste now, for she is probably able to follow instructions about rinsing and spitting out. When she has done her job and you have followed up with flossing, a final brushing, and rinsing, there are disclosing tablets or solution that can be used to see if any plaque (harmful film) or food remain. They are available without prescription and at low cost at pharmacies. The tablets and solution contain a dye made of vegetable coloring. Chewed by the child or used as a rinse, the dye leaves a stain on those teeth that are not yet clean. They should be brushed again carefully. It isn't necessary to go through this process at every brushing, but it would be worthwhile to at least consider it at the final brushing before bedtime each night.

Professional care—seeing the dentist for the first time—should be scheduled sometime between ages 2 and 3 years. A great deal depends on your child's maturity. Two-year-olds come with a wide range of personalities and capabilities. If you have a shy, clinging youngster who seems young for her age, do yourself and your dentist a favor and wait until she's 3. But if, on the other hand, your child is "2 going on 22," go ahead and sign her up for a professional check. Some dentists would rather not treat children younger than 3 years of age, so be sure to check with your dentist first.

Fears   Add to the fears discussed in Chapter 11 (water, animals, and vacuum cleaners) that 2-year-olds may be frightened by the sound of a flushing toilet, by dark colors, by large objects such as trains, or even by rain and wind. They may also fear separation at bedtime or at a parent's departure.

Pets and Playgrounds   A health hazard exists from pets that is both common and ignored. As much as 50 percent of cat feces, for example, is infected with toxoplasmosis. Although this parasitic disease usually causes only mild illness in adults, it can infect an unborn fetus much more seriously.

The danger from dog waste is just as serious, especially on public playgrounds, where as much as 25 percent of soil tested has been found to be infected with Toxocara, intestinal worms. This causes a disease in humans called toxocariasis, which can be mild—with only a mild fever and a rash—or serious, with neurological involvement and loss of vision. Children under age 4 years are the chief victims.

Pet birds and turtles also may be a problem. Psittacosis, also called parrot fever, causes flulike symptoms that require treatment with antibiotics. Pet turtles are commonly infected with the bacteria salmonella, which is fairly easily spread to humans, in whom it may cause salmonellosis, severe bacterial diarrhea. There is less danger from birds and turtles, of course, because they are a threat only in the households that own them. The danger from dogs and cats, on the other hand, is a threat to anyone who has young children and takes them to public playgrounds.

If you have a pet at home, have it checked regularly for the presence of disease. If you take your child to a public playground, watch her carefully to be sure she doesn't eat

316 ☆ THE BABY CHECKUP BOOK

dirt, and help her wash her hands thoroughly when she gets home.

Television   There are hair-raising statistics about children and television—that the average child will have watched hundreds of hours of television by the time she is a young adult, more hours than she spends in the classroom. It doesn't have to be that way. You can control the amount of time your child watches TV and you can also control what she watches.

You will probably want to limit your child's viewing, both in amount of time and subject matter. Whatever you decide—an hour a day or somewhat more—be consistent about enforcing it. For the younger child there are programs like *Sesame Street, Captain Kangaroo,* and *Mr. Rogers* to choose from. These are gentle, instructive programs that all young children enjoy. But even they can't take the place of a trip to the zoo, a walk in the park feeding the pigeons, or a half hour spent playing games with the letters of the alphabet. Even at its best, television can be a rather poor substitute for a real-life adventure.

In order to approve subject matter, you'll need to monitor what your child watches, and ideally, watch with her. Unless you are going to watch with your child and explain carefully that all the violence is make-believe, Saturday morning cartoons are not a very good choice for a 2-year-old. Or a 4- or 6-year-old either, for that matter. When one cartoon character plants a dynamite stick under another, doing no more damage than darkening his face and ruining his hat, somebody should explain that's not how it really is with dynamite. When a cartoon hero takes a pratfall off a 100-foot cliff and comes up smiling, you'd better hope your youngster doesn't think that's for real, either. Minute for minute, some of the most violent material on television appears on Saturday mornings.

Toys   Balls, blocks, push and pull toys, small trucks and cars without sharp edges or removable parts. Large, wheeled devices to ride on. Toy musical instruments are usually a big hit with this age group, particularly rhythm instruments like drums if you can stand it.

NEXT CHECKUP

Your child's next checkup will be in one year, when she is 3 years old. Between now and then, she will reach the following milestones in development, along with many others.

- Alternates feet going down stairs
- Does a broad jump
- Goes to the bathroom by self, is mostly dry at night
- Washes and dries own hands
- Dresses self completely with some help
- Recites and sings nursery rhymes and television commercials
- Plays with other children

EMERGENCY!

Telephone Number

Doctor _____

Poison Control Center _____

Pharmacy _____

Hospital _____

Ambulance/Aid Car _____

Fire Department _____

Police Department _____

_____

_____

_____

_____

_____

_____

_____

CHECKUP	EXAMINATION PROCEDURES
2–4 weeks	Repeat PKU test if first one done before baby was 72 hours old
2–3 months	Immunizations: DTP #1 (diphtheria/tetanus/pertussis) TOPV #1 (trivalent oral polio vaccine)
4–5 months	Immunizations: DTP #2 TOPV #2
6–7 months	Immunizations: DTP #3 TOPV #3 (optional)

CHECKUPS IN THE FIRST TWO YEARS

DEVELOPMENT	NUTRITION	REMINDERS (Anticipatory Guidance)
· Holds head up briefly · Follows object with eyes · May smile · Makes throaty noises	Milk	Watch urinary stream (boys) Acquire safe, approved baby equipment
· On tummy, lifts head · Relaxes fists · Smiles · Coos, laughs, and squeals	Milk	Safe handling, unsafe toys
· Improved head control · Rolls over one way · Smiles to get attention · Laughs out loud, vocalizes	Milk, small amounts of semisolid foods	Food allergy or intolerance Upper respiratory tract infections (URIs)
· Excellent head control · Sits (may need support) · Holds bottle/feeds self cracker · Babbles, imitates sounds	Milk, slightly lumpy foods	Childproofing the house

CHECKUP	EXAMINATION PROCEDURES
9–10 months	Hematocrit (Hct)/Hemoglobin (Hgb) blood test; cover test of eyes (optional)
1 year	Tuberculosis test
15 months	Immunizations: MMR/measles, mumps, rubella (German measles)
18 months	Immunizations: DTP #4 TOPV #4
2 years	Tuberculosis test Urinalysis (optional)

DEVELOPMENT	NUTRITION	REMINDERS (Anticipatory Guidance)
· Sits by self · Creeps · Shy with strangers · Says "Dada, Mama"	Three meals a day; reduce milk intake	Ear infections Community emergency resources Possible reduction of appetite
· Walks (alone or with one hand held) · Has thumb–finger (pincer) grasp · Drinks from cup · Says two or three words	Three meals a day, well-chopped table foods; milk limit 16 oz a day—in cup with meals	Setting limits (behavior)
· Walks · Stoops to pick up toy · Uses spoon · 3–10 words	If appetitie poor, reduce portions at meals, cut down on snacks	Fears, behavior
· Walks backward · Runs · Good with spoon and cup · 3–29 words	Three meals a day, same food as family	Toilet training, dental care
· Jumps · Kicks ball · Partly toilet-trained · 3–29 words	Table foods, no bottle	Negativism Temper tantrums Street and yard safety

GIRLS: BIRTH TO 36 MONTHS
PHYSICAL GROWTH
NCHS PERCENTILES*

NAME _____ RECORD # _____

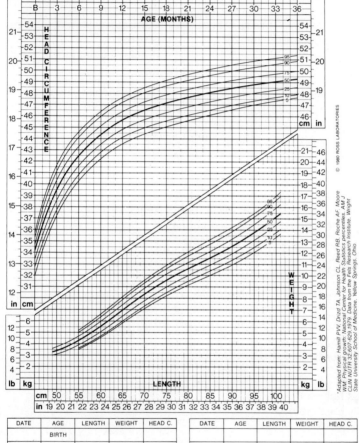

*Adapted from: Hamill PVV, Drizd TA, Johnson CL, Reed RB, Roche AF, Moore WM. Physical growth: National Center for Health Statistics percentiles. AM J CLIN NUTR 32:607-629 1979. Data from the Fels Research Institute, Wright State University School of Medicine, Yellow Springs, Ohio.

© 1980 ROSS LABORATORIES

DATE	AGE	LENGTH	WEIGHT	HEAD C.
	BIRTH			

DATE	AGE	LENGTH	WEIGHT	HEAD C.

Preferable to cow milk during the first year
SIMILAC® WITH IRON   **ADVANCE®**
Infant Formula   Nutritional Beverage

For milk-sensitivity
ISOMIL®
Soy Isolate Formula

ROSS LABORATORIES
COLUMBUS, OHIO 43216
DIVISION OF ABBOTT LABORATORIES, USA

G106 January 1980

☆ 324 ☆

**GIRLS: BIRTH TO 36 MONTHS
PHYSICAL GROWTH
NCHS PERCENTILES***

NAME _____ RECORD # _____

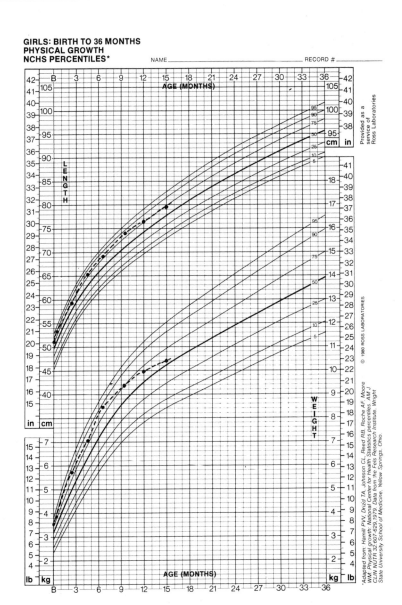

*Adapted from: Hamill PVV, Drizd TA, Johnson CL, Reed RB, Roche AF, Moore WM. Physical growth. National Center for Health Statistics percentiles. AM J CLIN NUTR 32:607-629, 1979. Data from the Fels Research Institute, Wright State University School of Medicine. Yellow Springs. Ohio.

Provided as a service of Ross Laboratories

© 1980 ROSS LABORATORIES

BOYS: BIRTH TO 36 MONTHS
PHYSICAL GROWTH
NCHS PERCENTILES*

NAME_____ RECORD # _____

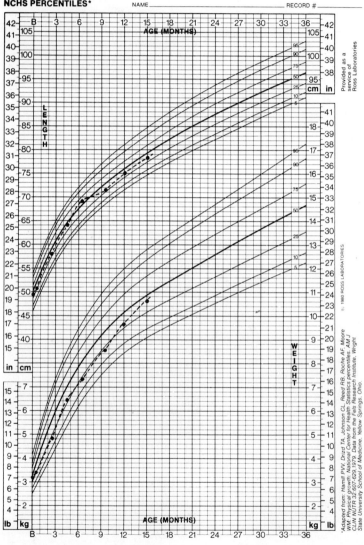

*Adapted from: Hamill PVV, Drizd TA, Johnson CL, Reed RB, Roche AF, Moore WM: Physical growth: National Center for Health Statistics percentiles. AM J CLIN NUTR 32:607-629,1979. Data from the Fels Research Institute, Wright State University School of Medicine, Yellow Springs, Ohio.

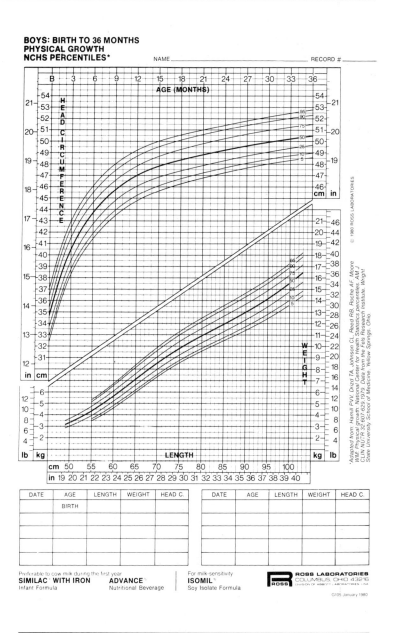

BOYS: BIRTH TO 36 MONTHS
PHYSICAL GROWTH
NCHS PERCENTILES*

NAME _____

RECORD # _____

IMMUNIZATION RECORD

Child's Name:		
Birth Date:		
Diphtheria/Tetanus/ Pertussis #1		
DTP #2		
#3		
#4		
Boosters		
Trivalent Oral Polio Vaccine		
#1		
TOPV #2		
#3		
Boosters		
Measles/Mumps/ Rubella		
MMR		

BIBLIOGRAPHY

GENERAL PEDIATRICS

American Academy of Pediatrics. *Standards of Child Health Care*. 2d. ed. Evanston: American Academy of Pediatrics, 1972.

American Academy of Pediatrics. *Standards and Recommendations for Hospital Care of Newborn Infants*. 6th ed. Evanston: American Academy of Pediatrics, 1977.

Nelson, Waldo E., M.D., ed. *Textbook of Pediatrics*. 11th ed. Philadelphia: W. B. Saunders Company, 1979.

Smith, David W., M.D. *Introduction to Clinical Pediatrics*. 2d ed. Philadelphia: W. B. Saunders Company, 1977.

Waring, William W., M.D., and Louis O. Jeansonne III, M.S., M.D. *Practical Manual of Pediatrics: A Pocket Reference for Those Who Treat Children*. Saint Louis: The C. V. Mosby Company, 1975.

CHILD DEVELOPMENT

Brazelton, T. Berry. *Infants and Mothers*. New York: Dell Publishing Co., 1972.

Brazelton, T. Berry. *Toddlers and Parents*. New York: Dell Publishing Co., Inc., 1976.

Burck, Frances Wells. *Babysense: A Practical and Supportive Guide to Baby Care*. New York: St. Martin's Press, 1979.

Caplan, Frank. *The First Twelve Months of Life*. New York: Bantam Books, Inc., 1978.

Caplan, Frank and Caplan, Theresa. *The Second Twelve Months of Life*. New York: Bantam Books, Inc., 1980.

Erickson, Marcene L., R.N. *Assessment and Management of Developmental Changes in Children*. St. Louis: The C. V. Mosby Company, 1976.

Illingworth, R. S., M.D. *The Development of the Infant and*

Young Child. 7th ed. Edinburgh: Churchill Livingstone, 1980.

Knobloch, Hilda, M.D, Dr.P.H. *Manual of Developmental Diagnosis: The Administration and Interpretation of the Revised Gesell and Amatruda Developmental and Neurologic Examination.* Hagerstown: Harper & Row, 1980.

Spock, Benjamin. *Baby and Child Care.* New York: Pocket Books, 1981.

White, Burton L. *The First Three Years of Life.* New York: Avon Books, 1978.

IMMUNIZATIONS

American Academy of Pediatrics. *Report of the Committee on Infectious Diseases.* 11th ed. Evanston: American Academy of Pediatrics, 1977.

NUTRITION

American Academy of Pediatrics. *Pediatric Nutrition Handbook.* Evanston: American Academy of Pediatrics, 1979.

La Leche League. *The Womanly Art of Breastfeeding. 1981. Available through LLL leaders. See page 52.*

Pipes, Peggy L., R.D., M.P.H.. *Nutrition in Infancy and Childhood.* 2d ed. St. Louis: The C. V. Mosby Company, 1981.

Pryor, Karen. *Nursing Your Baby,* New York: Pocket Books, 1980

THE PHYSICAL EXAMINATION

Gundy, John H., M.D. *Assessment of the Child in Primary Health Care.* New York: McGraw-Hill Book Company, 1981.

Hillman, Robert S., M.D.; Brian W. Goodell, M.D.; Scott M. Grundy, M.D., Ph.D.; James R. McArthur, M.D.; and

James H. Moller, M.D. *Clinical Skills: Interviewing, History Taking and Physical Diagnosis.* New York: McGraw-Hill Book Company, 1981.

SAFETY AND FIRST AID

Hillman, Sheilah, and Robert S. Hillman, M.D. *Traveling Healthy: A Complete Guide to Medical Services in 23 Countries.* New York: Penguin Books, 1980.
McIntire, Matilda S., M.D., ed. *Handbook on Accident Prevention.* Hagerstown: Harper & Row, 1980.

PUBLISHED PAPERS BY THE AMERICAN ACADEMY OF PEDIATRICS

Committee on Drugs, Committee on Fetus and Newborn. 1980. Prophylaxis and Treatment of Neonatal Gonococcal Infections. *Pediatrics* 65: 1047–48.
Committee on Environmental Hazards. 1976. Effects of Cigarette Smoking on the Fetus and Child. *Pediatrics* 57: 411–13.
Committee on Environmental Hazards. 1972. Lead Content of Paint Applied to Surfaces Accessible to Young Children. *Pediatrics* 49: 918–21.
Committee on Fetus and Newborn. 1979. Care of the Newborn in the Delivery Room. *Pediatrics* 64: 970.
Committee on Fetus and Newborn. 1971. Oxygen Therapy in the Newborn Infant. *Pediatrics* 47: 1086–87.
Committee on Fetus and Newborn. 1975. Report of the Ad Hoc Task Force on Circumcision. *Pediatrics* 56: 610–11.
Committee on Fetus and Newborn. 1974. Skin Care of Newborns. *Pediatrics* 54: 682–83.
Committee on Infant and Preschool Child. 1972. The Sudden Infant Death Syndrome. *Pediatrics* 50: 964–65.
Committee on Nutrition (with the Nutrition Committee of the Canadian Pediatric Society). 1978. Breast Feeding: A Commentary in Celebration of the International Year of the Child. *Pediatrics* 62: 591–601.

Committee on Nutrition. 1976. Commentary on Breast-Feeding and Infant Formulas, Including Proposed Standards for Formulas. *Pediatrics* 57: 278–85.

Committee on Nutrition. 1971. Correspondence Re Iron Fortified Formulas. *Pediatrics* 48: 152–56.

Committee on Nutrition. 1980. On the Feeding of Supplemental Food to Infants. *Pediatrics* 65: 1178–81.

Committee on Nutrition. 1972. Fluoride as a Nutrient. *Pediatrics* 49: 456–60.

Committee on Nutrition. 1979. Fluoride Supplementation: Revised Dosage Schedule. *Pediatrics* 63: 150–52.

Committee on Nutrition. 1971. Iron Fortified Formula. *Pediatrics* 47: 786.

Committee on Nutrition. 1976. Iron Supplementation for Infants. *Pediatrics* 58: 765–68.

Committee on Nutrition. 1977. Nutritional Aspects of Vegetarianism, Health Foods, and Fad Diets. *Pediatrics* 59: 460–64.

Committee on Nutrition. 1971. Vitamin K Supplementation for Infants Receiving Milk Substitute Infant Formulas and for Those with Fat Malabsorption. *Pediatrics* 48: 483–87.

Committee on Pediatric Aspects of Physical Fitness, Recreation, and Sports. 1980. Swimming Instructions for Infants. *Pediatrics* 65: 847.

OTHER PUBLICATIONS

Bayley, Nancy. *Manual for the Bayley Scales of Infant Development.* New York: The Psychological Corporation, 1969.

Calott, Anne, et al. *Dental Care for Children with Heart Disease.* American Heart Association, 1979.

Cobo, Edgard, M.D. 1973. Effect of Different Doses of Ethanol on the Milk-Ejecting Reflex in Lactating Women. *Am. J. Obstet. Gynecol.* 115: 817–21.

Feldman, Kenneth W., M.D. 1980. Prevention of Childhood Accidents: Recent Progress. *Pediatr. Rev.* 2: 75–82.

Frankenburg, William K., M.D. et al. *Denver Developmental Screening Test,* revised 1975 ed.

Geffner, Mitchell E., M.D.; Darleen R. Powars, M.D.; and William T. Choctar, M.D. 1981. Acquired Methemoglobinemia. *West J. Med.* 134: 7–10.

Kahn, Alice, R.N.R. 1981. A Parents' Guide to Children's Ear Infections. *Medical Self-Care* Spring: 48–50.

Keating, James P., M.D. 1973. Infantile Methemoglobinemia Caused by Carrot Juice. *N. Engl. J. Med.* 288: 824–26.

Little, Ruth E., Sc.D.; Francia A. Shultz, M.S.W.; and Wallace Mandell, Ph.D., M.P.H. 1976. Drinking During Pregnancy. *J. Stud. Alcohol* 37: 375–79.

Milani and Comparetti. *Milani Comparetti Motor Development Screening Test.* Omaha: Meyer Children's Rehabilitation Institute, 1977.

Mofenson, Howard C., M.D. et al. 1981. Baby Powder—A Hazard! *Pediatrics* 68: 265–66.

Moss, Arthur, J., M.D. 1981. Blood Pressure in Infants, Children and Adolescents. *West. J. Med.* 134: 296–314.

United States Department of Health, Education, and Welfare. *Smoking and Health: A Report of the Surgeon General.* Washington, D.C.: U.S. Government, 1979.

ABOUT THE AUTHOR

Sheilah Hillman lives in Cape Elizabeth, Maine with her husband, Robert, a doctor and a medical consultant for this book. They have two grown children. A graduate of Tufts University, she has worked as a newspaper reporter, book editor, public relations consultant, and journalism teacher. The Hillmans are co-authors of *Traveling Healthy: A Complete Guide to Medical Services in 23 Countries,* published in 1980.

ABOUT THE CONSULTANTS

James H. Moller, M.D. is a professor of pediatrics at the University of Minnesota in Minneapolis and Dwan Professor for Research in Education in Pediatric Cardiology. Past chairman of the Minnesota Chapter of the American Academy of Pediatrics, he lives with his wife in Minneapolis. They have two children.
Robert S. Hillman, M.D. is chief of medicine at the Maine Medical Center in Portland and professor of medicine at the University of Vermont in Burlington. He was until recently a professor of medicine at the University of Washington in Seattle and director of the university's Health Sciences Learning Resources Center.

ABOUT THE PHOTOGRAPHER

Michael McIntosh is a staff photographer of the Medical Photography Unit at the University of Washington Health Sciences Learning Resources Center in Seattle. He is married and the father of two sons, ages 9 years and 9 months.

ABOUT THE ILLUSTRATORS

Trese Rand is a Northwest illustrator who specializes in eye surgery and children's open heart surgery. She lives on a farm in Bellevue, Washington. Dale Leuthold and Phyllis J. Wood, both members of the Association of Medical Illustrators (A.M.I.), are on the medical illustration staff of the University of Washington Health Sciences Learning Resources Center in Seattle.

22